ECG Interpretation

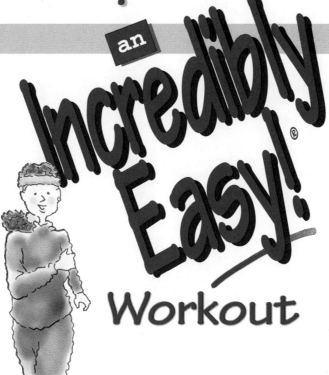

an Incredibly Easy!® Workout

ECG Interpretation

an

Incredibly Easy!®

Workout

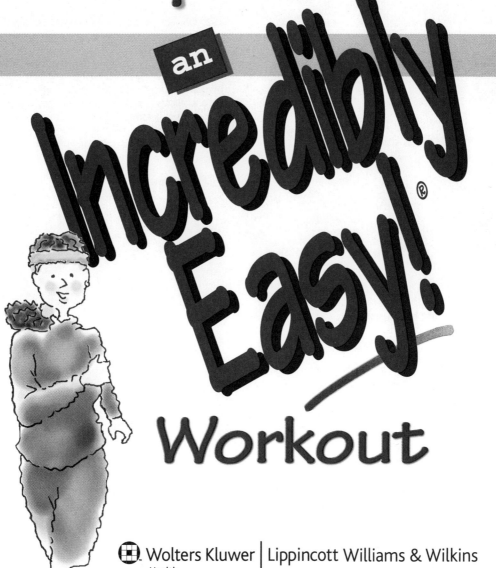

Wolters Kluwer | Lippincott Williams & Wilkins
Health

Philadelphia · Baltimore · New York · London
Buenos Aires · Hong Kong · Sydney · Tokyo

Staff

Executive Publisher
Judith A. Schilling McCann, RN, MSN

Editorial Director
David Moreau

Clinical Director
Joan M. Robinson, RN, MSN

Art Director
Mary Ludwicki

Senior Managing Editor
Jaime Stockslager Buss, MSPH, ELS

Editors
Kristin Baum; Gale Thompson, RN, BA; Susan Williams

Copy Editors
Kimberly Bilotta (supervisor), Dorothy P. Terry,
Pamela Wingrod

Designer
Lynn Foulk

Illustrator
Bot Roda

Digital Composition Services
Diane Paluba (manager), Joyce Rossi Biletz,
Donna S. Morris

Associate Manufacturing Manager
Beth J. Welsh

Editorial Assistants
Karen J. Kirk, Jeri O'Shea, Linda K. Ruhf

Workout regimen

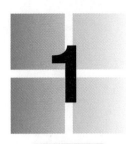

Cardiac anatomy and physiology

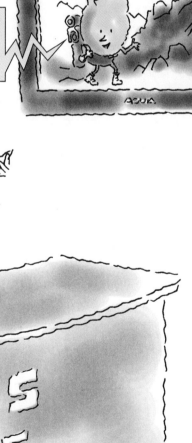

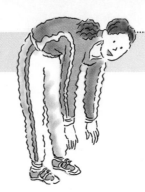

Cardiac anatomy and physiology review

The heart's valves

■ *Tricuspid*—Atrioventricular (AV) valve between the right atrium and right ventricle
■ *Mitral*—AV valve between the left atrium and left ventricle
■ *Aortic*—semilunar valve between the left ventricle and aorta
■ *Pulmonic*—semilunar valve between the right ventricle and pulmonary artery

Blood flow

■ Deoxygenated blood from the body ▶ right atrium ▶ right ventricle ▶ lungs (where it's oxygenated) ▶ left atrium ▶ left ventricle ▶ aorta and the body

Coronary arteries and veins

■ *Right coronary artery*—supplies blood to the right atrium and ventricle and part of the left ventricle
■ *Left anterior descending artery*—supplies blood to the anterior wall of the left ventricle, interventricular septum, right bundle branch, and left anterior fasciculus of the left bundle branch
■ *Circumflex artery*—supplies blood to the lateral walls of the left ventricle, left atrium, and left posterior fasciculus of the left bundle branch
■ *Cardiac veins*—collect blood from the capillaries of the myocardium
■ *Coronary sinus*—returns blood to the right atrium

Cardiac cycle dynamics

■ *Atrial kick*—atrial contraction, contributes about 30% of cardiac output
■ *Cardiac output*—amount of blood the heart pumps in 1 minute, equal to heart rate times stroke volume
■ *Stroke volume*—amount of blood ejected with each ventricular contraction; affected by preload, afterload, and contractility
 – *Preload*—passive stretching exerted by blood on the ventricular muscle at the end of diastole
 – *Afterload*—amount of pressure the left ventricle must work against to pump blood into the aorta
 – *Contractility*—ability of the heart muscle cells to contract after depolarization

Innervation of the heart

■ *Sympathetic nervous system*—increases heart rate, automaticity, AV conduction, and contractility through release of norepinephrine and epinephrine
■ *Parasympathetic nervous system*—vagus nerve stimulation reduces heart rate and AV conduction through release of acetylcholine

Transmission of electrical impulses

Generation and transmission of electrical impulses depend on:
■ *Automaticity*—cell's ability to spontaneously initiate an impulse, such as found in pacemaker cells
■ *Excitability*—cell's response to an electrical stimulus
■ *Conductivity*—cell's ability to transmit an electrical impulse to another cardiac cell
■ *Contractility*—how well the cell contracts after receiving a stimulus

Depolarization-repolarization cycle

Cardiac cells undergo the following cycles of depolarization and repolarization as impulses are transmitted:
■ *Phase 0: Rapid depolarization*—cell receives an impulse from a nearby cell and is depolarized
■ *Phase 1: Early repolarization*—early rapid repolarization occurs
■ *Phase 2: Plateau phase*—period of slow repolarization
■ *Phase 3: Rapid repolarization*—cell returns to original state
■ *Phase 4: Resting phase*—cell rests and readies itself for another stimulus

Cardiac conduction

■ Electrical impulse route: Sinoatrial (SA) node ▶ internodal tracts and Bachmann's bundle ▶ AV node ▶ bundle of His along the bundle branches ▶ Purkinje fibers

Intrinsic firing rates

■ *SA node*—60 to 100/minute
■ *AV junction*—40 to 60/minute
■ *Purkinje fingers*—20 to 40/minute

Abnormal impulses

■ *Automaticity*—cardiac cell's ability to initiate an impulse on its own
■ *Retrograde conduction*—impulses are transmitted backward toward the atria
■ *Reentry*—impulse follows a circular conduction path

■ Batter's box

Before jumping into the workout, let's see if you can run the course on key cardiac concepts. Fill in the blanks with the appropriate words. *Hint:* One word is used more than once.

Cardiac stats

The heart is located behind the _____ , between the _____ and
₁ ... ₂

in front of the spine. The base of the heart lies just below the _____ rib. The
₃

apex tilts forward and down, toward the _____ side of the body.
₄

The heart's wall is comprised of three layers. The outer layer, or _____ , is
₅

made up of squamous _____ cells. The _____ is the middle
₆ ... ₇

layer and makes up the _____ part of the heart's wall. The final, innermost
₈

layer is called the _____ . It contains _____ tissue with bundles
₉ ... ₁₀

of smooth muscle.

    The heart contains _____ chambers (two _____ and two
₁₁ ... ₁₂

_____) and four _____ (two _____ valves and
₁₃ ... ₁₄ ... ₁₅

two _____ valves).
₁₆

Get your circulation going

Deoxygenated blood from the body returns to the heart through the inferior and superior

_____ and empties into the right _____ . From there, blood
₁₇ ... ₁₈

flows through the _____ into the _____ ventricle, which pumps
₁₉ ... ₂₀

blood into the _____ . Then blood returns to the left atrium and flows to the
₂₁

left ventricle. Oxygenated blood is pumped to the _____ and the body by
₂₂

the left ventricle.

Options

aorta

atria

atrioventricular

atrium

endocardium

endothelial

epicardium

epithelial

four

largest

left

lungs

mediastinum

myocardium

right

second

semilunar

tricuspid valve

vena cavae

ventricles

valves

■■
■ Finish line

Label each layer of the heart.

1. _____

2. _____

3. _____
4. _____
5. _____

■■
■ Strike out

Some of the following statements about the layers of the heart are incorrect. Cross out the incorrect statements.

1. The serous pericardium has three layers.

2. The myocardium makes up the largest portion of the heart's wall.

3. The pericardium is a tough, protective sac that surrounds and protects the heart.

4. The parietal layer adheres to the surface of the heart.

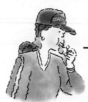

Coaching session
How the heart changes with age

As a person ages, even the healthiest heart becomes slightly smaller and loses its contractile strength and efficiency. By age 70, cardiac output at rest has diminished by 30% to 35%. As the myocardium becomes more irritable, extra systoles, sinus arrhythmias, and sinus bradycardias may occur. Increased fibrous tissue may also infiltrate the sinoatrial node and internodal atrial tracts, causing atrial fibrillation and flutter.

Time to flex those muscles! Push yourself to the limit with this challenge.

Cross-training

Complete this crossword puzzle to really give your knowledge of cardiac anatomy and physiology a workout.

Across

1. This valve is located where the left ventricle meets the aorta.

4. High-pressure work determines the _____ of a chamber's walls.

6. The interventricular _____ separates the ventricles and helps them to pump.

7. Another term for cusps is _____.

10. Damage to chordae tendineae may result in backward blood flow, causing a heart _____.

11. The arteries supply _____ blood to the body.

Down

2. Backflow from one chamber to another is called _____.

3. This valve is located between the left atrium and left ventricle.

4. The mitral valve has _____ cusps.

5. This term collectively describes the pulmonic and aortic valves.

8. The types of atrioventricular valves are mitral and _____.

9. The chordae tendineae anchor the _____ to the papillary muscles in the heart wall.

Pep talk

"Champions know there are no shortcuts to the top. They climb the mountain one step at a time."
—Judi Adler

■ Finish line

The illustration below shows the anatomy of a normal heart. Label all of the components.

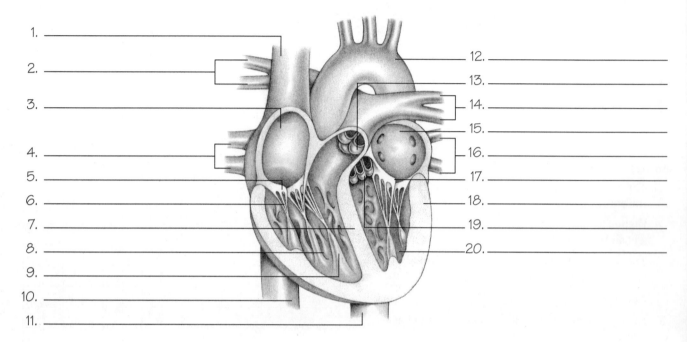

1. _____
2. _____
3. _____
4. _____
5. _____
6. _____
7. _____
8. _____
9. _____
10. _____
11. _____

12. _____
13. _____
14. _____
15. _____
16. _____
17. _____
18. _____
19. _____
20. _____

■ Jumble gym

Unscramble the words at left to discover terms related to the heart and surrounding vessels.
Then use the circled letters to form a word that correctly answers the question below.

Question: Valves open and close in response to what kind of changes in the chambers they connect?

1. T C E L V S I E N R _ _ _ _ ○ _ _ _ _ ○

2. A E N E V E V A C A _ ○ _ _ _ _ _ _ _ ○

3. O N Y R C A O R N I S U S _ _ ○ _ _ _ _ _ ○ _ _ _ _

4. S P U C S _ ○ _ ○ _

Answer: _ _ _ _ _ _ _

> Get in shape with this cardiac conundrum.

■■
■ You make the call

Here's a chance to review how blood flows through the heart while also brushing up on cardiac anatomy. Follow the path of blood flow through the heart by circling the term that correctly completes each statement.

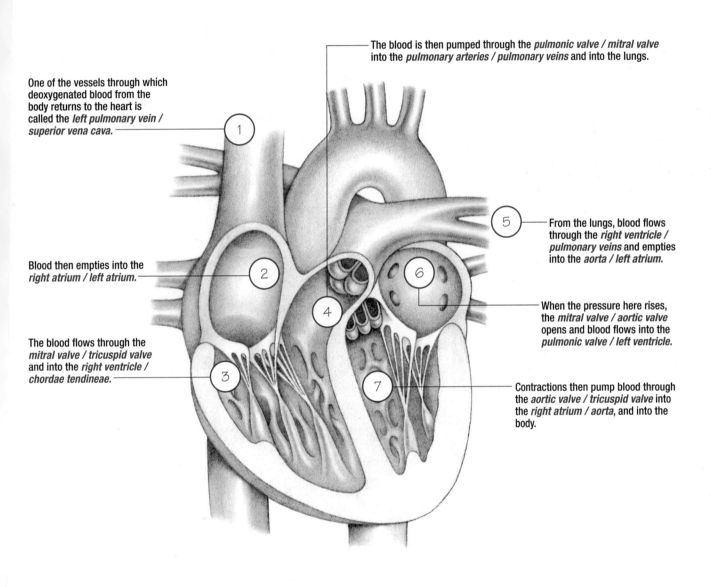

The blood is then pumped through the *pulmonic valve / mitral valve* into the *pulmonary arteries / pulmonary veins* and into the lungs.

One of the vessels through which deoxygenated blood from the body returns to the heart is called the *left pulmonary vein / superior vena cava.*

From the lungs, blood flows through the *right ventricle / pulmonary veins* and empties into the *aorta / left atrium.*

Blood then empties into the *right atrium / left atrium.*

When the pressure here rises, the *mitral valve / aortic valve* opens and blood flows into the *pulmonic valve / left ventricle.*

The blood flows through the *mitral valve / tricuspid valve* and into the *right ventricle / chordae tendineae.*

Contractions then pump blood through the *aortic valve / tricuspid valve* into the *right atrium / aorta*, and into the body.

8

■■
■ You make the call

Label the five phases of the cardiac cycle below and describe what happens during each phase.

1. _____

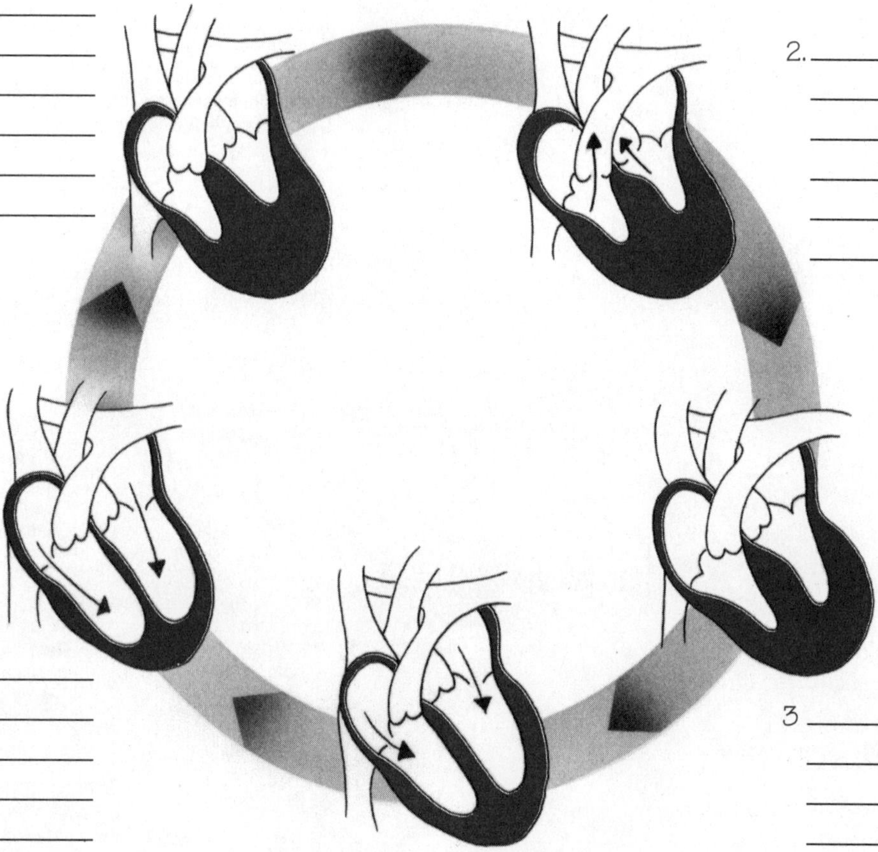

_____

_____

_____

_____

_____

2. _____

_____

_____

_____

_____

5. _____

_____

_____

_____

_____

_____

3. _____

_____

_____

_____

_____

4. _____

_____

_____

_____

_____

With all my cycles, you can call me Lance Heartstrong!

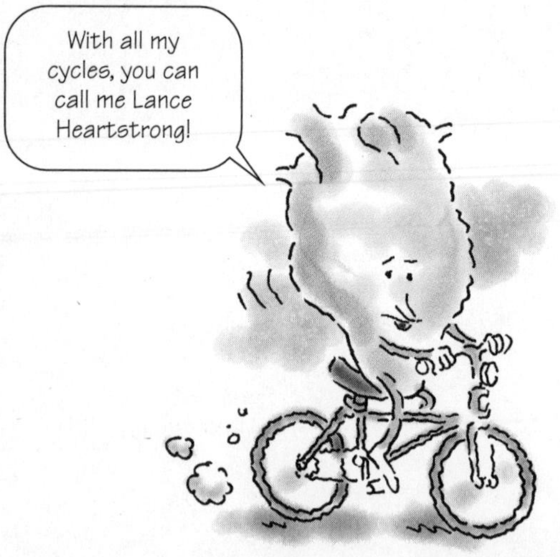

■ Hit or miss

Some of the following statements about cardiac physiology are true; the others are false. Label each one accordingly.

_____ 1. Atrial kick contributes to 30% of cardiac output.

_____ 2. Cardiac output is the amount of blood the heart pumps in 5 minutes.

_____ 3. Three factors affect stroke volume: preload, afterload, and myocardial contractility.

_____ 4. Contractility is the ability of muscle cells to contract after depolarization.

_____ 5. Preload is the amount of pressure the left ventricle must work against to pump blood into circulation.

■ Jumble gym

Unscramble the words at left to decode terms relating to cardiac dynamics.
Then use the circled letters to form a word that correctly answers the question below.

Question: Preload is determined by the pressure and amount of blood remaining in the left ventricle at the end of what phase of the cardiac cycle?

1. Amount of blood ejected with each ventricular contraction

O E K T R S M O L V E U ◯ _ _ ◯ _ _ _ _ ◯ _ _ _

2. The sum of the processes that occur during one heartbeat

D C A C R I A L Y C E C _ _ _ ◯ _ _ _ _ _ _ _ ◯

3. Also known as *atrial kick*

A T L I A R S L Y S O T E _ _ _ ◯ _ _ _ _ _ ◯ _ _ _

4. Pressure the left ventricle must work against to pump blood into the aorta

F O L R A D A T E _ _ _ _ _ _ _ ◯ _

Answer: _ _ _ _ _ _ _ _

■ You make the call

Using the space provided, describe how sodium, calcium, and potassium are affected during each of the phases of the depolarization and repolarization cycle.

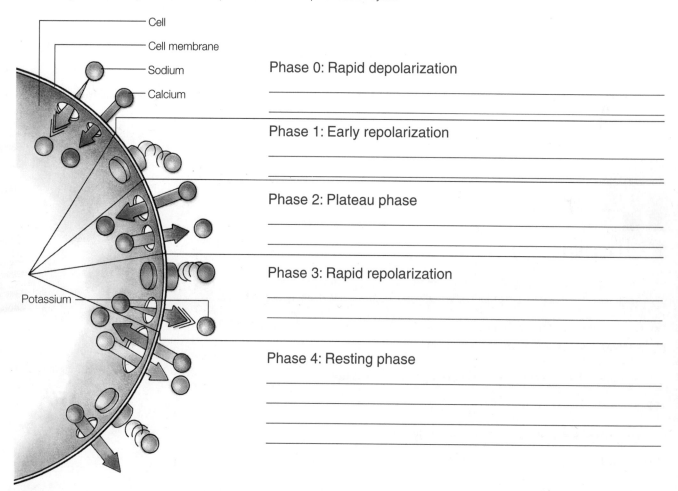

Cell

Cell membrane

Sodium

Calcium

Potassium

Phase 0: Rapid depolarization

_____

_____

Phase 1: Early repolarization

_____

_____

Phase 2: Plateau phase

_____

_____

Phase 3: Rapid repolarization

_____

_____

Phase 4: Resting phase

_____

_____

_____

_____

■ Match point

Match each of the phases of the depolarization and repolarization cycle on the left with its correct description on the right.

1. Phase 0 _____
2. Phase 1 _____
3. Phase 2 _____
4. Phase 3 _____
5. Phase 4 _____

A. A period of slow repolarization occurs during this phase.

B. The cell receives an impulse from a neighboring cell and is depolarized.

C. This is the resting phase. The cell is ready for another stimulus.

D. Early, rapid repolarization occurs.

E. This is a phase of rapid repolarization as the cell returns to its original state.

■ Strike out

Some of the following statements about the heart's nerve supply are incorrect. Cross out the incorrect statements.

1. The parasympathetic nervous system is the heart's accelerator.

2. The sympathetic branch of the nervous system is also called the adrenergic system.

3. Acetylcholine increases heart rate, automaticity, atrioventricular conduction, and contractility.

4. Carotid sinus massage activates baroreceptors, which can slow a rapid heart rate.

■ Hit or miss

Some of the following statements are true; the others are false. Label each one accordingly.

_____ 1. Afterload is the pressure needed from the ventricles to overcome higher pressure in the aorta.

_____ 2. Preload is the passive stretching exerted by blood on the ventricular muscle at the end of systole.

_____ 3. Starling's law says that the less the cardiac muscles stretch in diastole, the more forcefully they contract in systole.

_____ 4. The vagus nerve carries impulses that slow heart rate and the conduction of impulses.

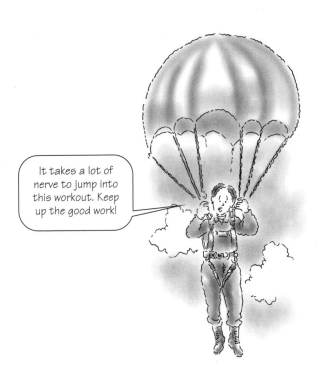

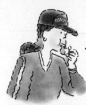

Coaching session
Action potential

As impulses are transmitted, cardiac cells undergo cycles of depolarization and repolarization. After a stimulus occurs, ions cross the cell membrane and cause an action potential, or cell depolarization. An action potential curve shows the electrical changes that occur in a myocardial cell during the depolarization-repolarization cycle. This graph shows the changes in a non-pacemaker cell.

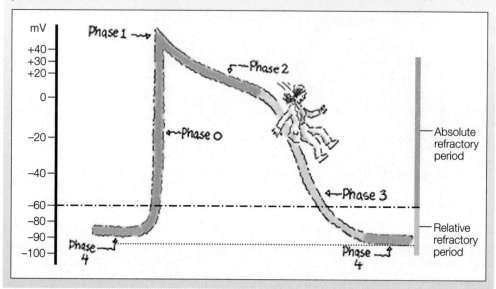

Match point

Match each of the characteristics of cardiac cells on the left with the correct term on the right.

1. Ability to transmit an electrical impulse to another cardiac cell _____

2. How well a cell responds to an electrical stimulus _____

3. Ability to spontaneously initiate an impulse _____

4. How well a cell contracts after receiving a stimulus _____

A. Contractility

B. Excitability

C. Conductivity

D. Automaticity

Jumble gym

Unscramble each word to discover terms related to the depolarization-repolarization cycle.
Then use the circled letters to form a word that correctly answers the question below.

Question: **The cell membrane becomes impermeable to sodium during which phase of the depolarization-repolarization cycle?**

1. OLPEAIZDR _ _ _ _ ◯ _ _ ◯ _

2. IPUELMS ◯ _ _ _ _ ◯ _

3. TOCNIA IPOTLETAN RCVUE
   _ _ ◯ _ _ _   _ _ _ _ ◯ _ _ _ _   _ _ _ _ _

4. GVLTAEO _ _ _ _ _ ◯ _

Answer: _ _ _ _ _ _ _

With all of this stimulation, it feels good to finally be in my resting phase.

Starting lineup

Place the steps of impulse conduction in the correct order.

The impulse travels to the bundle of His.	1.
The impulse is delayed at the AV node.	2.
The SA node generates an impulse.	3.
The impulse travels along the right and left bundle branches.	4.
	5.
The impulse travels through the atria along Bachmann's bundle and the internodal pathways.	6.
The impulse reaches the Purkinje fibers that conduct it rapidly through the heart muscle.	

Finish line

Label the heart's pacemaker cells with their names and intrinsic firing rates.

1. _____
   _____

2. _____
   _____

3. _____
   _____

Train your brain

Sound out each group of pictures and symbols to reveal a statement about one of the heart's pacemakers.

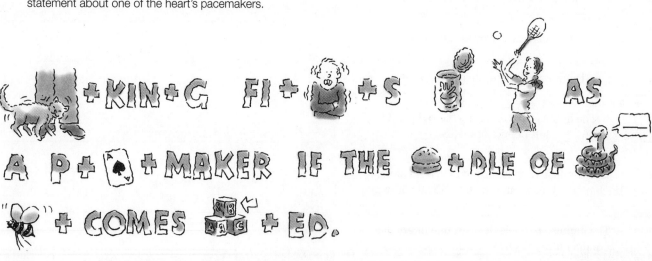

■■
■ Strike out

Some of the following statements about abnormal impulses are incorrect. Cross out the incorrect statements.

1. A decrease in automaticity of cells in the sinoatrial node can cause bradycardia.

2. Early afterdepolarization can be caused by hypercalcemia.

3. Reentry events are impulses that depolarize twice in a row and at a faster-than-normal rate.

4. Impulses that transmit backward take longer than normal and can cause out-of-synch beats.

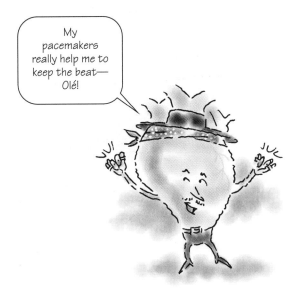

■■
■ Match point

Match each of the characteristics of abnormal impulse conduction on the left with the correct term on the right.

1. Repetitive ectopic firings caused by secondary depolarization _____

2. Depolarization that occurs after the cell has been fully repolarized _____

3. Compensatory beat generated by a lower pacemaker site _____

4. Possible result of partial depolarization _____

A. Delayed afterdepolarization

B. Secondary depolarization

C. Triggered activity

D. Escape rhythm

■ Cross-training

Complete the crossword puzzle using the clues below.

Across

2. The stretching of muscle fibers in the ventricles
4. Characteristic of pacemaker cells that generate impulses without being stimulated
5. Displays the heart's electrical activity
6. Term used to describe cardiac cells at rest
7. Phase 2 of the depolarization-repolarization cycle
9. Another term for backward conduction
11. Contributes 30% of the cardiac output (_____ kick)
12. Characteristic of cardiac cells resulting from ion shifts across the cell membrane
13. Term that describes when an impulse follows a circular conduction path

Down

1. Activated by carotid sinus massage
3. Cardiac output = heart rate × _____ volume
8. Caused by an increase or decrease in cell's automaticity
10. Fibers that conduct impulses rapidly to assist in depolarization and contraction

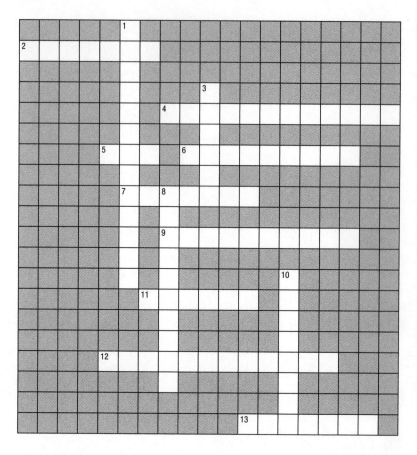

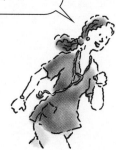

Stay motivated. You're almost at the finish line for this chapter!

Match point

Match each type of conduction on the left with the appropriate image on the right.

1. Premature impulse _____

2. Reentry _____

3. Unidirectional _____

A.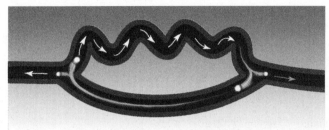

B.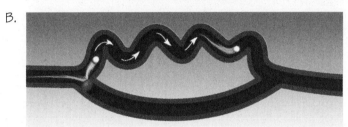

C.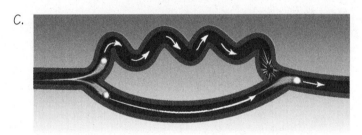

Hit or miss

Some of the following statements about abnormal impulses are true; the others are false. Label each one accordingly.

_____ 1. Automaticity is a special characteristic of Purkinje fibers that generates impulses automatically.

_____ 2. If a cell's automaticity is increased or decreased, an arrhythmia can occur.

_____ 3. Impulses that begin below the AV node can be transmitted backward toward the ventricles.

_____ 4. Impulses can sometimes cause depolarization twice in a row at a faster-than-normal rate, an event known as reentry.

_____ 5. An injured pacemaker cell may partially depolarize, rather than fully depolarize, leading to spontaneous or secondary depolarization.

■■ ■ Odd man out

In each of the word groupings below, circle the odd man out (the word that doesn't belong) by figuring out the connection among all of the other words in the group.

1. Heart   Lungs   Blood vessels   Lymphatics

2. Pericardium   Epicardium   Endocardium   Myocardium

3. Atria   Mediastinum   Ventricles

4. Bicuspid   Tricuspid   Mitral   Pulmonic

5. Arteries   Venules   Veins   Arterioles   Alveoli   Capillaries

6. Systemic   Intrinsic   Coronary   Pulmonary

■■ ■ Circuit training

Trace the path of blood from the heart to the lungs and back again by drawing arrows between the boxes below.

| Arteries |

| Right ventricle | | Pulmonary arteries | | Arterioles | | Lung capillaries |

| Pulmonary valve |

| Pulmonary veins | | Venules | | Alveoli |

| Left atrium |

| Veins |

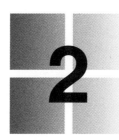

2

Obtaining a rhythm strip

Wow, is he lacking direction?! His rhythm is weak, he's wandering, and he's got interference. He can't be a winner without understanding how a lead functions. Are you grounded in the basics? Let's see if you can pedal through this chapter.

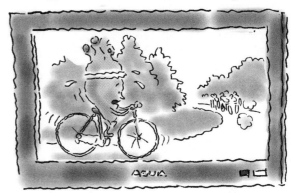

SPORTS NITE

Obtaining a rhythm strip review

Leads and planes

- *Lead*—View of the heart's electrical activity between a positive and negative pole
  - When electrical current travels toward the negative pole, the waveform deflects mostly downward
  - When current travels toward the positive pole, the waveform deflects mostly upward
- *Plane*—Cross-section view of the heart's electrical activity
  - Frontal plane, a vertical cut through the middle of the heart, provides an anterior-posterior view
  - Horizontal plane, a transverse cut through the middle of the heart, provides a superior or inferior view

Types of ECGs

- *12-lead ECG* records electrical activity from 12 heart views
- *Single-lead* or *dual-lead monitoring* provides continuous cardiac monitoring

12-lead ECG

- Six limb leads provide information about the heart's frontal (vertical) plane
- Bipolar leads (I, II, and III) require a negative and positive electrode for monitoring
- Unipolar leads (aV_R, aV_L, and aV_F) record information from one lead and require only one electrode
- Six precordial leads (leads V_1 through V_6) provide information about the heart's horizontal plane

Leads I, II, and III

- Typically produce positive deflection on ECG tracings
- Lead I helps monitor atrial arrhythmias and hemiblocks
- Lead II commonly aids in routine monitoring and detecting of sinus node and atrial arrhythmias
- Lead III helps detect changes associated with inferior wall myocardial infarction

Precordial leads

- Lead V_1
  - Biphasic
  - Distinguishes right and left ventricular ectopic beats
  - Monitors ventricular arrhythmias, ST-segment changes, and bundle-branch blocks
- Leads V_2 and V_3
  - Biphasic
  - Monitor ST-segment elevation
- Lead V_4
  - Produces a biphasic waveform
- Lead V_5
  - Produces a positive deflection on the ECG
  - Can show changes in the ST-segment or T wave (when used with Lead V_4)
- Lead V_6
  - Produces a positive deflection on the ECG

Modified leads

- Lead MCL_1
  - Similar to V_1
  - Assesses QRS-complex arrhythmias, P-wave changes, and bundle-branch defects.
  - Monitors premature ventricular beats
  - Distinguishes different types of tachycardia
- Lead MCL_6
  - Similar to V_6
  - Monitors ventricular conduction changes

Electrode configurations

- *Three-electrode system* uses one positive electrode, one negative electrode, and a ground
- *Five-electrode system* uses four stationary leads and an exploratory chest lead to monitor modified chest leads

ECG strip

- 1 small horizontal block = 0.04 second
- 5 small horizontal blocks = 1 large block = 0.20 second
- 5 large horizontal blocks = 1 second
- Normal strip = 30 large horizontal blocks = 6 seconds
- 1 small vertical block = 0.1 mV
- 1 large vertical block = 0.5 mV
- Amplitude (mV) = number of small blocks from baseline to highest or lowest point

Monitoring problem causes

- *Artifact*—excessive movement or dry electrode causes baseline to appear wavy, bumpy, or tremulous
- *Interference*—electrical power leakage, interference from other equipment, or improper equipment grounding produces a thick, unreadable baseline
- *Wandering baseline*—chest wall movement, poor electrode placement, or poor electrode contact causes an undulating baseline
- *Faulty equipment*—faulty and worn equipment can cause monitoring problems and place the patient at risk for shock

■■ ■ Batter's box

See if you can hit one out of the ballpark by filling in the blanks with the appropriate words.

Current events

The heart's _____ activity produces currents that radiate through the
₁

surrounding _____ to the _____ . When _____
₂ ₃ ₄

are attached to the skin, they sense those currents and transmit them to an

_____ monitor. The currents are then transformed into _____
₅ ₆

that represent the heart's _____ - _____ cycle.
₇ ₈

ECG overview

An ECG shows the precise sequence of electrical events occurring in the

_____ cells. It allows the nurse to monitor phases of myocardial
₉

_____ and to identify _____ and _____
₁₀ ₁₁ ₁₂

disturbances. A series of ECGs can be used as a _____ comparison to
₁₃

assess cardiac _____ .
₁₄

Leads (plane and simple)

The ECG records information about the waveforms from two perspectives:

_____ and _____ . The lead provides a view of the heart's
₁₅ ₁₆

electrical activity between one _____ pole and one _____
₁₇ ₁₈

pole. The _____ plane gives an anterior-to-posterior view of the heart's
₁₉

electrical activity. The _____ plane gives a superior or an inferior view of the heart.
₂₀

Options

baseline

cardiac

conduction

contraction

depolarization

electrical

electrocardiogram

electrodes

frontal

function

horizontal

leads

negative

planes

positive

repolarization

rhythm

skin

tissue

waveforms

Match point

Match each of the terms on the left with its correct definition on the right.

1. Frontal plane _____

2. Plane _____

3. Lead's axis _____

4. Lead _____

A. Provides a view of the heart's electrical activity between one positive pole and one negative pole

B. Refers to the direction of current moving through the heart

C. A vertical cut through the middle of the heart providing an anterior or posterior view of electrical activity

D. A cross-sectional perspective of the heart's electrical activity

You make the call

Describe what's happening to the direction of electrical currents shown.

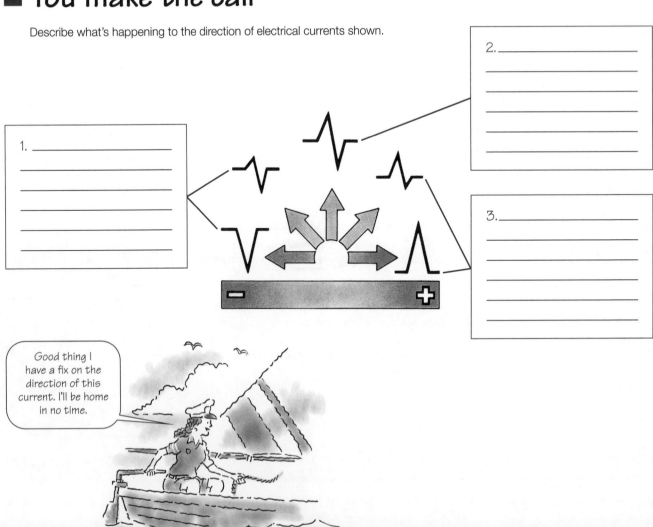

1. _____

2. _____

3. _____

Good thing I have a fix on the direction of this current. I'll be home in no time.

Jumble gym

Use the clues to help you unscramble words related to leads and planes.
Then use the circled letters to form a word that correctly answers the question.

Question: **What term is used to describe a waveform that goes in both directions?**

1. Name for a waveform on which no electrical activity occurs

ECILRCIOEST $\bigcirc$ _ _ _ _ _ $\bigcirc$ _ _ _ _

2. The visual representation of electrical current on an ECG

FVMOAWESR _ _ _ _ $\bigcirc$ _ _ _ $\bigcirc$

3. Type of comparison for which a series of ECGs can be used to assess cardiac rhythm

NLSEBEIA $\bigcirc$ _ _ _ _ $\bigcirc$ _ _

4. Name for a transverse cut through the middle of the heart that provides either a superior or an inferior view

TZOLHIARON NPELA $\bigcirc$ _ _ _ _ _ _ _ _ $\bigcirc$ _ _ _ _

Answer: _ _ _ _ _ _ _ _

Strike out

Some of the following statements about ECG leads are incorrect. Cross out the incorrect statements.

1. Augmented leads record information from one lead and are unipolar.

2. The abbreviation MCL stands for "modified cardiac lead."

3. The six limb leads include leads V_1, V_2, V_3, V_4, V_5, and V_6.

4. The six precordial leads provide information about the heart's horizontal plane.

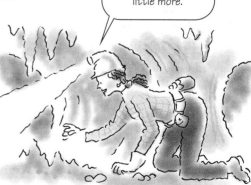

Need more light shed on the subject of leads? Let's explore them a little more.

■ Hit or miss

Some of the following statements are true; the others are false. Label each one accordingly.

_____ 1. Leads I, II, and III are unipolar.

_____ 2. A 12-lead ECG records information by placing electrodes on the limbs and the chest.

_____ 3. The six limb leads provide information about the heart's frontal plane.

_____ 4. Continuous information about the heart's electrical activity can be achieved through single-lead or dual-lead monitoring.

_____ 5. The two leads that are most commonly monitored simultaneouly in dual-lead monitoring are leads I and V_1.

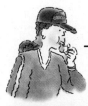

Coaching session

Hardwire monitoring vs. telemetry

Hardwire monitoring, where electrodes are connected directly to the cardiac monitor, provides a continuous cardiac rhythm display and transmits the ECG tracing to a console at the nurses' station. It can also track pulse oximetry, blood pressure, hemodynamic measurements, and other parameters through various attachments to the patient. It does have drawbacks, however, that include limited patient mobility, patient discomfort, the possibility of lead disconnection (and loss of cardiac monitoring), and accidental shock to the patient (rare).

Telemetry monitoring frees the patient from cumbersome wires, but it still requires skin electrodes. It's especially useful for detecting arrhythmias that occur at rest or during sleep, exercise, or stressful situations. Most telemetry systems can monitor only heart rate and rhythm.

■ Cross-training

Complete the crossword puzzle by using the clues below.

Across

4. Direction of waveform deflection as current travels toward a negative pole

6. The six V leads

7. Type of information about the heart's electrical activity single-lead or dual-lead monitoring provides

8. Term to describe waveform line appearance when no activity or weak activity occurs

11. Type of cut the frontal plane makes through the middle of the heart

12. The "F" in aV_F

13. Term used to describe the precordial leads that are placed in sequence across a patient's chest

Down

1. Type of unipolar lead

2. Requires a negative and positive electrode for monitoring

3. Plane that provides a superior or inferior view

5. Direction a waveform deflects as current travels toward the positive pole

9. Type of monitoring system that allows more patient activity

10. The lead's axis (the _____ of the current moving through the heart)

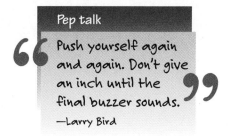

Pep talk

" Push yourself again and again. Don't give an inch until the final buzzer sounds. "
—Larry Bird

■■
■ Strike out

Some of the following statements about monitoring are incorrect. Cross out the incorrect statements.

1. Limited patient mobility is a drawback to telemetry monitoring.

2. Hardwire monitors also have the ability to track pulse oximetry, blood pressure, and hemodynamic measurements.

3. Telemetry monitoring is useful for detecting arrhythmias that occur during exercise.

4. Hardwire monitoring is generally used in step-down units and medical-surgical units.

■■
■ Finish line

Label the leads and electrodes for Einthoven's triangle.

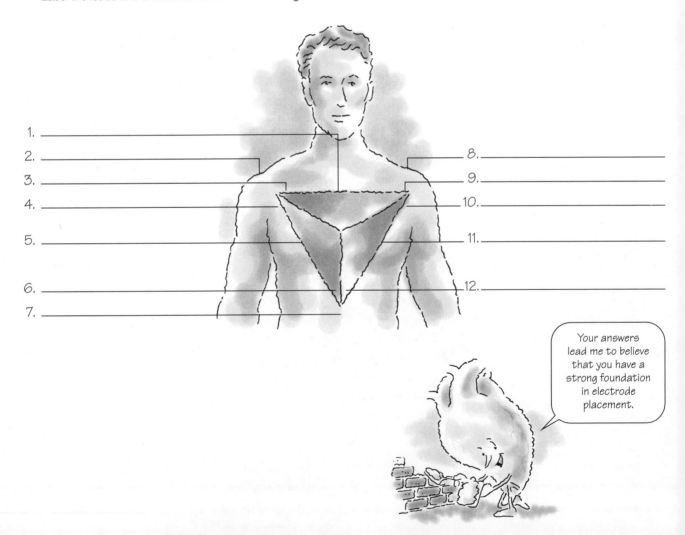

1. _____
2. _____
3. _____
4. _____
5. _____
6. _____
7. _____

8. _____
9. _____
10. _____
11. _____
12. _____

Your answers lead me to believe that you have a strong foundation in electrode placement.

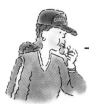

Coaching session
Augmented leads

Leads aV_R, aV_L, and aV_F are called *augmented leads.* They measure electrical activity between one limb and a single electrode. Lead aV_R provides no specific view of the heart. Lead aV_L shows electrical activity coming from the heart's lateral wall. Lead aV_F shows electrical activity coming from the heart's inferior wall.

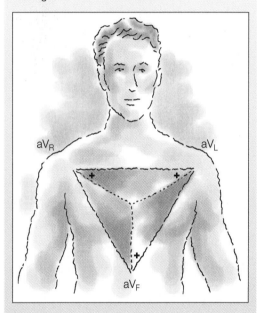

■ Match point

Match the electrode location on the left with the appropriate lead on the right.

1. Positive electrode on the left leg; negative electrode on the right arm _____

2. Positive electrode in the fourth intercostal space to the right of the sternum; negative electrode on the left upper chest _____

3. Positive electrode on the left leg; negative electrode on the left arm _____

4. Positive electrode on the left arm; negative electrode on the right arm _____

A. Lead III

B. Lead I

C. MCL_1

D. Lead II

■ Hit or miss

Some of the following statements are true; the others are false. Label each one accordingly.

_____ 1. Lead I is helpful in monitoring atrial rhythms and hemiblocks.

_____ 2. Lead aV_L provides no specific view of the heart.

_____ 3. Lead III is useful in detecting changes associated with an inferior wall myocardial infarction.

_____ 4. Augmented leads produce a positive, high-voltage deflection, resulting in tall P, R, and T waves.

■ Match point

Match the six precordial leads on the left with their appropriate electrode placement on the right.

1. Lead V_1 _____

2. Lead V_2 _____

3. Lead V_3 _____

4. Lead V_4 _____

5. Lead V_5 _____

6. Lead V_6 _____

A. Placed at the fifth intercostal rib space at the left midclavicular line

B. Placed at the fifth intercostal rib space at the left midaxillary line

C. Placed on the right side of the sternum at the fourth intercostal rib space

D. Placed to the left of the sternum at the fourth intercostal rib space

E. Placed at the fifth intercostal space at the left anterior axillary line

F. Placed between V_2 and V_4

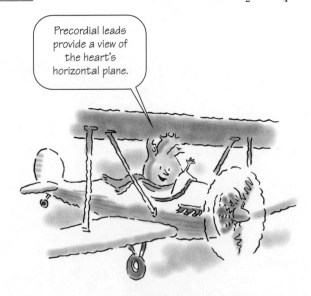

Precordial leads provide a view of the heart's horizontal plane.

Jumble gym

Unscramble the letters to find terms related to ECG leads. Then use the circled letters to form a word that correctly answers the question below.

Question: What kind of conduction change does lead MCL_6 monitor?

1. P N I A R U L O _ _ ◯ _ _ ◯ _ _

2. T E L C L E R C I A V T Y C I A I T ◯ _ _ _ _ _ ◯ _ _   _ _ _ _ ◯ _ _ _

3. R T E R U N C _ ◯ _ _ _ ◯

4. D P O A R C E I L R _ ◯ _ _ _ _ _ ◯ _

5. N T O O R I M _ _ ◯ _ _ ◯

Answer: _ _ _ _ _ _ _ _ _ _ _

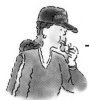

Coaching session
Applying electrodes

- Wash the application site with soap and water.
- Briskly rub the area with the special rough patch on the back of the electrode, a dry washcloth, or a gauze pad. Be sure not to damage the skin.
- Clip dense hair at the electrode site, if needed.
- Remove the backing on the pregelled electrode, making sure it's moist. If the electrode is dry, discard it and select another.
- Press one side of the electrode against the patient's skin, pull gently, and then press the opposite side of the electrode against the skin.
- Using two fingers, press the adhesive edge around the outside of the electrode to the patient's chest.

■ Match point

Match the electrode positions for the leads of a telemetry system with the correct illustration.

1. Lead I _____
2. Lead II _____
3. Lead III _____
4. Lead MCL$_1$ _____
5. Lead MCL$_6$ _____

A.
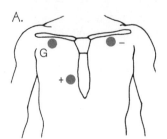

B.
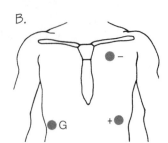

C.
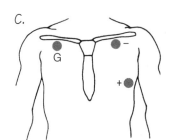

D.
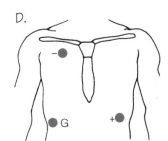

E.
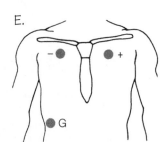

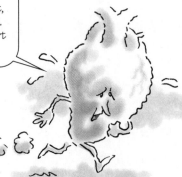

It's great to get in a good workout, but take my lead. Monitor your heart rate carefully.

■ Strike out

Some of the following statements about electrode systems are incorrect. Cross out the incorrect statements.

1. The three-electrode system is the only one that doesn't use a ground electrode.

2. The five-electrode system can monitor any one of six modified chest leads as well as the standard limb leads.

3. Wires that attach to the electrodes in the five-electrode system are usually color-coded to help in placement.

4. The four-electrode system has a left leg electrode that becomes a permanent ground for all leads.

■ Finish line

Label each leadwire and its corresponding color in the five-leadwire system.

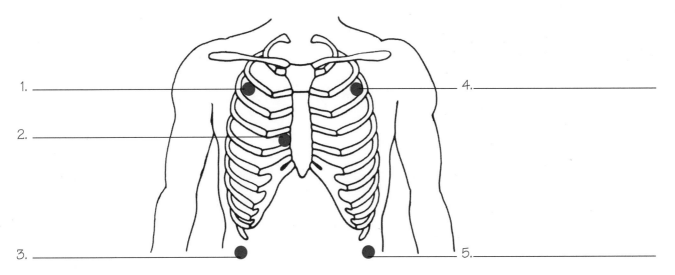

1. _____

2. _____

3. _____

4. _____

5. _____

Starting lineup

Put the following electrode placement steps in the order they should be performed.

Choose electrode placement sites for the chosen lead.	1.
Prepare the patient's skin.	2.
Apply the electrode.	3.
Explain the electrode placement to the patient.	4.
If needed, clip dense hair closely at each site.	5.

Hit or miss

Some of the following statements are true; the others are false. Label each one accordingly.

_____ 1. A clip-on leadwire should be applied after the electrode has been secured to the patient's skin.

_____ 2. Electrodes should be removed from the patient's skin and replaced with new electrodes every 48 hours.

_____ 3. Electrodes should never be placed over soft tissue.

_____ 4. Patients with oily skin should have their skin cleaned with an alcohol pad before electrode placement.

■■
■ Cross-training

Complete the crossword puzzle by using the clues below.

Across

1. Adjust this dial if a waveform appears too high or too low on the screen.
5. Adjust this control if a waveform appears too large or too small on the screen.
6. An ECG strip's vertical axis measures this length in millimeters.
7. The _____ control on the monitor can produce a printout of the patient's cardiac rhythm.
9. Count the number of small blocks from the _____ to the highest or lowest point of the wave, segment or interval to determine amplitude.

Down

2. Another name for an ECG strip is _____ .
3. Electrical voltage is measured in _____ .
4. The horizontal axis of the ECG strip represents _____ .
6. Heart rate _____ are generally set 10 to 20 bpm higher and lower than the patient's heart rate.
8. To verify that each heartbeat is being detected, compare the patient's _____ rate with the rate on the monitor.

■■
■ Jumble gym

Unscramble the letters to find terms related to ECG monitoring. Then use the circled letters to form a word that correctly answers the question below.

Question: What kind of detector do some monitors have that generates a rhythm strip automatically whenever the heart rate alarm goes off?

1. RINOGOMTIN YTSESM ◯_ _ _ _ _ _◯_ _   _◯_ _ _ _

2. ICRDACA HMYHTR _ _◯_ _ _ _   _◯_ _ _ _

3. BATAHERET ◯_ _ _ _ _ _ _◯

4. CVILRATE IXSA _ _◯_ _ _◯_   ◯_ _ _

Answer: _ _ _ _ _ _ _ _ _ _

■ Strike out

Some of the following statements about ECGs are incorrect. Cross out the incorrect statements.

1. Wandering baseline appears on the ECG as a baseline that's thick and unreadable.

2. Faulty equipment can cause accidental shocks to the patient.

3. Artifact interference is also called 60-cycle interference.

4. The baseline of an artifact ECG appears wavy, bumpy, or tremulous.

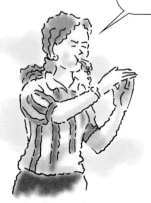

Interference due to improperly grounded equipment. Penalty of 60 cycles!

■ Match point

Match the ECG monitoring problem on the left with the illustration that represents this problem.

1. Artifact _____

2. False high-rate alarm _____

3. Weak signals _____

4. Wandering baseline _____

5. Fuzzy baseline _____

6. Baseline (no waveform) _____

A.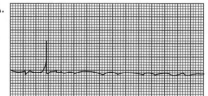

B.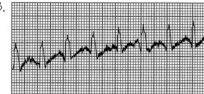

C.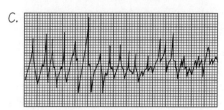

D.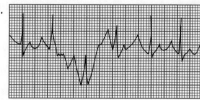

E.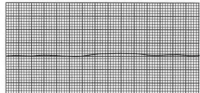

F.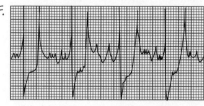

3

Interpreting a rhythm strip

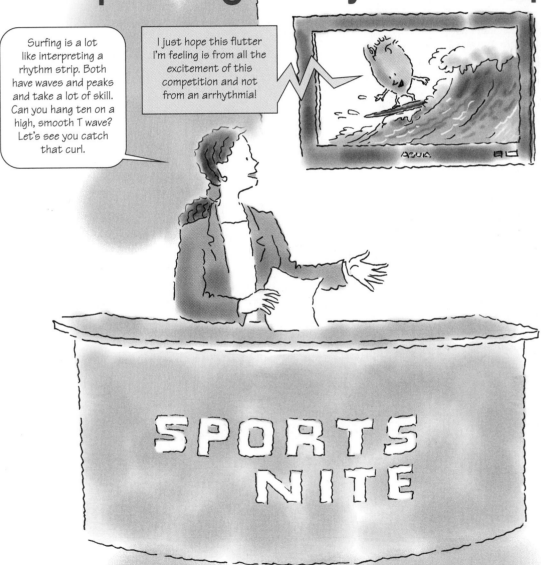

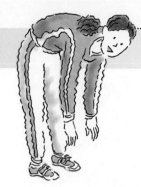

Interpreting a rhythm strip review

ECG components

Normal P wave
- *Location*—before the QRS complex
- *Amplitude*—2 to 3 mm high
- *Duration*—0.06 to 0.12 second
- *Configuration*—usually rounded and upright
- *Deflection*—positive or upright in leads I, II, aV$_F$, and V$_2$ to V$_6$; usually positive but may vary in leads III and aV$_L$; negative or inverted in lead aV$_R$; biphasic or variable in lead V$_1$

Normal PR interval
- *Location*—from the beginning of the P wave to the beginning of the QRS complex
- *Duration*—0.12 to 0.20 second

Normal QRS complex
- *Location*—follows the PR interval
- *Amplitude*—5 to 30 mm high but differs for each lead used
- *Duration*—0.06 to 0.10 second, or half the PR interval
- *Configuration*—consists of the Q wave, the R wave, and the S wave
- *Deflection*—positive in leads I, II, III, aV$_L$, aV$_F$, and V$_4$ to V$_6$ and negative in leads aV$_R$ and V$_1$ to V$_3$

Normal ST segment
- *Location*—from the S wave to the beginning of the T wave
- *Deflection*—usually isoelectric; may vary from – 0.5 to +1 mm in some precordial leads

Normal T wave
- *Location*—after the S wave
- *Amplitude*—0.5 mm in leads I, II, and III and up to 10 mm in the precordial leads
- *Configuration*—typically round and smooth
- *Deflection*—usually upright in leads I, II, and V$_3$ to V$_6$; inverted in lead aV$_R$; variable in all other leads

Normal QT interval
- *Location*—from the beginning of the QRS complex to the end of the T wave
- *Duration*—varies; usually lasts from 0.36 to 0.44 second

Normal U wave
- *Location*—after T wave
- *Configuration*—typically uprights and rounded
- *Deflection*—upright

Interpreting a rhythm strip: 8-step method
- Step 1: Determine the rhythm
- Step 2: Determine the rate
- Step 3: Evaluate the P wave
- Step 4: Measure the PR interval
- Step 5: Determine the QRS complex duration
- Step 6: Examine the T waves
- Step 7: Measure the QT interval
- Step 8: Check for ectopic beats and other abnormalities

Normal sinus rhythm

Normal sinus rhythm is the standard against which all other rhythms are compared.

Characteristics
- Regular rhythm
- Normal rate
- P wave for every QRS complex; all P waves similar in size and shape
- Normal PR intervals
- All QRS complexes similar in size and shape
- Normal T waves
- Normal QT intervals

Match point

Match the part of the ECG complex from the column on the left with the appropriate illustration on the right.

1. P wave _____

2. PR interval _____

3. QRS complex _____

4. ST segment _____

5. T wave _____

6. QT interval _____

7. U wave _____

A.
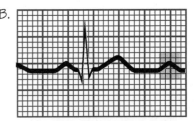

B.

C.
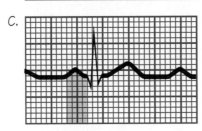

D.
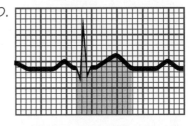

E.
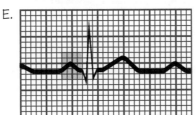

F.
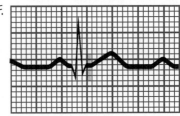

G.
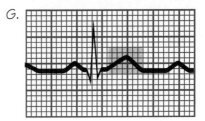

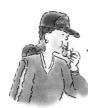

Coaching session
Normal sinus rhythm

Get yourself up to speed by reviewing the characteristics of normal sinus rhythm:

• Atrial and ventricular rhythms are regular.

• Atrial and ventricular rates fall between 60 and 100 beats/minute, the SA node's normal firing rate, and all impulses are conducted to the ventricles.

• P waves are rounded, smooth, and upright in lead II, signaling that a sinus impulse has reached the atria.

• The PR interval is normal (0.12 to 0.20 second), indicating that the impulse is following normal conduction pathways.

• The QRS complex is of normal duration (less than 0.12 second), representing normal ventricular impulse conduction and recovery.

• The T wave is upright in lead II, confirming that normal repolarization has taken place.

• The QT interval is within normal limits (0.36 to 0.44 second).

• No ectopic or aberrant beats occur.

■ Batter's box

Review a few key concepts about interpreting ECGs by filling in the blanks below with the appropriate words. *Hint:* Some answer options are used more than once.

Have a complex?

An ECG complex represents the _____ events occurring in one
                                        1

_____ cycle. A complex consists of five waveforms labeled with the letters
         2

_____ , _____ , _____ , _____ , and
         3   4   5   6

_____ . ECG tracings represent the conduction of _____
         7   8

_____ from the _____ to the _____ .
         9   10   11

Find the rhythm

To determine the heart's atrial and ventricular rhythms, use the _____ method
                                                                          12

or the _____ method. For atrial rhythm, measure the _____
              13   14

between consecutive _____ waves. To determine the ventricular rhythm,
                             15

measure the intervals between consecutive _____ waves in the QRS
                                                   16

complexes.

Check the rate

To establish atrial and ventricular heart rates, use the _____ method if the
                                                                 17

heart rhythm is regular. The _____ method is the easiest way to calculate rate,
                                     18

whereas the _____ method requires that you memorize a set of numbers.
                    19

Options

10-times

1,500

atria

caliper

cardiac

electrical

impulses

intervals

P

paper-and-pencil

Q

R

S

sequence

T

ventricles

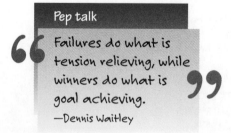

Pep talk

Failures do what is tension relieving, while winners do what is goal achieving.
—Dennis Waitley

■■
■ Finish line

Identify the components of a normal ECG waveform on the illustration below.

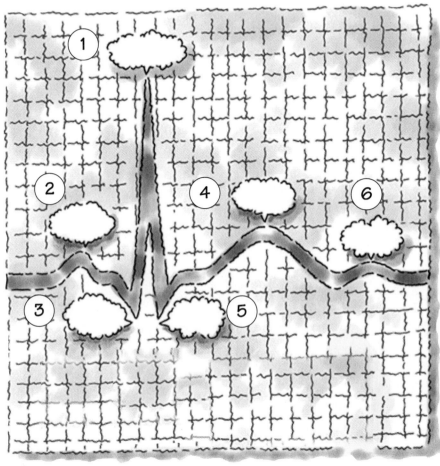

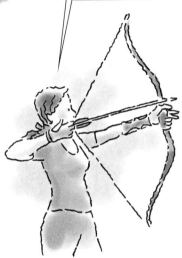

Now that you're loosened up, see if you can hit the mark in a few more games.

■ Strike out

Some of the following statements about the components of ECGs are incorrect. Cross out the incorrect statements.

1. Infants and children have faster heart rates than adults, producing long PR and QRS intervals.

2. No P wave with the QRS complex may indicate hypercalcemia.

3. The U wave represents the recovery period of the Purkinje or ventricular conduction fibers.

4. A prolonged QT interval increases the risk of torsades de points, a life-threatening arrhythmia

5. In older adults, the QRS axis shifts to the right.

6. The T wave represents repolarization of the ventricles.

■ Hit or miss

Some of the following statements are true; the others are false. Label each one accordingly.

_____ 1. Peaked, notched, or enlarged P waves may represent retrograde conduction from the atrioventricular junction toward the atria.

_____ 2. Changes to the PR interval indicate an altered impulse formation or a conduction delay.

_____ 3. The P wave is usually rounded and upright.

_____ 4. A notched R wave may represent myocardial infarction.

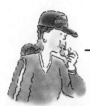

Coaching session
ECGs in older adults

Keep the patient's age in mind when interpreting an ECG. ECG changes in older adults include increased PR, QRS, and QT intervals, decreased amplitude of the QRS complex, and a shift of the QRS axis to the left.

Jumble gym

Use the clues to help you unscramble words related to ECG complexes. Then use the circled letters to form a word that correctly answers the question.

Question: What's one type of P wave that signifies conduction by a route other than the sinoatrial node?

1. Direction of a waveform

N E E L C T F O I D __ __ __ __ ⚪ __ __ __ __ __

2. Term for a complex containing both an upward and downward deflection

S H I C B P A I ⚪ __ __ __ __ ⚪ __ __

3. Height of a waveform

P L A M D T U E I ⚪ __ __ __ __ __ __ __ __

4. Transmission of an electrical impulse

N U D C I C O T O N __ __ ⚪ __ __ __ ⚪ __ __ __

Answer: __ __ __ __ __ __

You make the call

Closely monitoring the ST segments on a patient's ECG can help you detect ischemia or injury before infarction develops. Describe what's occurring in the ST segments shown here.

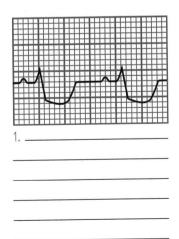

1. _____
_____
_____
_____
_____

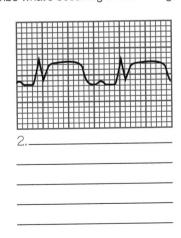

2. _____
_____
_____
_____
_____

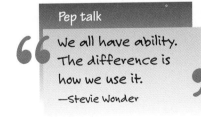

■ Boxing match

Fill in the answers to the clues below by using all of the syllables in the box. The number of syllables for each answer is shown in parentheses. Use each syllable only once. The first answer has been provided for you as an example.

AM	~~E~~	~~EL~~	DE	DE
FLEC	GRADE	IZA	LAR	P
PLI	PO	RET	RO	TION
~~TION~~	TION	TUDE	~~VA~~	WAVE

1. Distance above the baseline
   (4) E L E V A T I O N

2. Response of a myocardial cell to an electrical impulse
   (5) _ _ _ _ _ _ _ _ _ _ _ _ _ _

3. Height of a waveform
   (3) _ _ _ _ _ _ _ _

4. Direction of a waveform, based on the direction of a current
   (3) _ _ _ _ _ _ _ _ _

5. Depolarization that occurs backward
   (3) _ _ _ _ _ _ _ _ _

6. Deflection that represents atrial activity
   (2) _ _ _ _ _

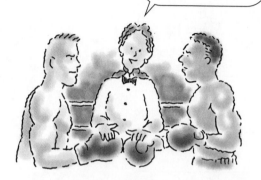

Ready for a quick boxing match? Put on your thinking cap and, remember, no jabs below the waist.

▪▪ Starting lineup

Put the following rhythm strip analysis steps in the order in which they should be performed.

Determine the duration of the PR interval.	1.
Determine the rate.	2.
Evaluate any other components.	3.
Determine the rhythm.	4.
Determine the duration of the QRS complex.	5.
Evaluate the T waves.	6.
Evaluate the P wave.	7.
Determine the duration of the QT interval.	8.

▪▪ Hit or miss

Some of the following statements are true; the others are false. Label each one accordingly.

_____ 1. The 10-times method is the easiest way to calculate heart rate.

_____ 2. To get the atrial rate using the sequence method, first find a T wave that peaks on a heavy black line.

_____ 3. The 1,500 method should be used for irregular heart rhythms.

_____ 4. To determine the atrial rate for the 10-times method, obtain a 6-second strip, count the number of P waves, and multiply by 10.

You make the call

Using the space provided, describe the characteristics of this rhythm strip. Then interpret the rhythm.

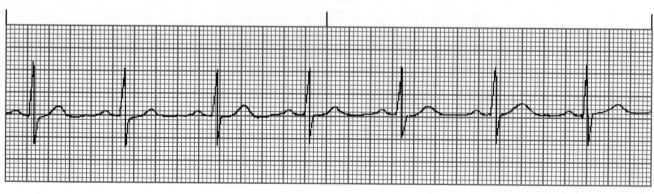

Atrial rhythm: _____

Ventricular rhythm: _____

Atrial rate: _____

Ventricular rate: _____

P wave: _____

PR interval: _____

QRS complex: _____

T wave: _____

QT interval: _____

Other: _____

Interpretation: _____

■ Cross-training

Complete the following crossword puzzle to test your knowledge of ECG interpretation terms.

Across

4. A pulse is created by this ventricular activity.

6. This parameter should always be checked to correlate it with the heart rate on the ECG.

7. The P wave represents atrial _____ .

8. Rapid rate calculation is also called the _____ method.

Down

1. When evaluating a QRS complex, special attention should be paid to the _____ and configuration.

2. If an ST segment is 1 mm or more above the baseline, it's considered _____ .

3. These PR intervals indicate that the impulse started somewhere other than the sinoatrial node.

5. The QRS complex represents intraventricular _____ time.

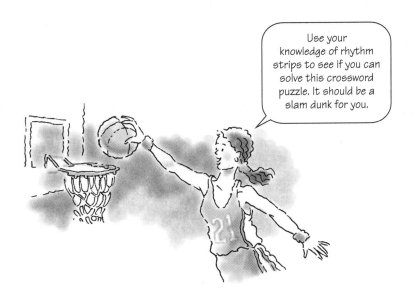

Use your knowledge of rhythm strips to see if you can solve this crossword puzzle. It should be a slam dunk for you.

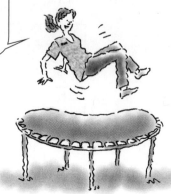

By now, you must have a lot of ECG information bouncing around in your head. Let's put it to use with some ECG interpretation.

■ You make the call

Using the space provided, describe the characteristics of this rhythm strip. Then interpret the rhythm.

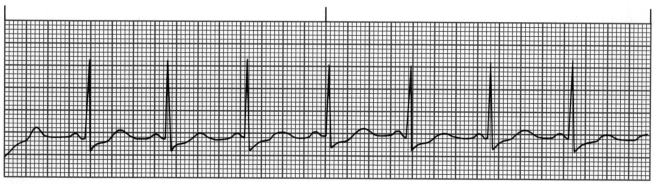

Atrial rhythm: _____

Ventricular rhythm: _____

Atrial rate: _____

Ventricular rate: _____

P wave: _____

PR interval: _____

QRS complex: _____

T wave: _____

QT interval: _____

Other: _____

Interpretation: _____

■■ ■ Train your brain

Sound out each group of pictures and symbols to reveal a statement about one of the ECG's waveforms.

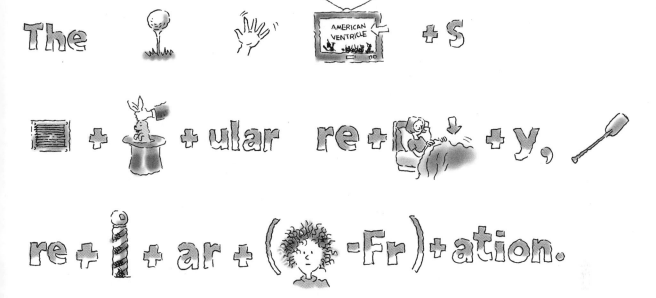

■■ ■ Strike out

Some of the following statements about ECGs are incorrect. Cross out the incorrect statements.

1. The J point marks the end of the QRS complex and the beginning of the ST segment.

2. The slower the heart rate, the shorter the QT interval.

3. Bumps in a T wave may indicate that a U wave is hidden in it.

4. The U wave may not appear on an ECG.

5. Pointed or heavily notched T waves in an adult may indicate pericarditis.

6. When documenting a QRS complex, uppercase letters should be used to indicate a wave with an amplitude greater than 3 mm.

■ Match point

Match the ECG interpretation step on the left with the correct technique on the right.

1. Determining the duration of QT interval _____
2. Determining the ventricular rhythm _____
3. Determining the atrial rate with 10-times method _____
4. Determining the duration of the PR interval _____

A. Multiply the number of small squares between the start of the P wave and the start of the QRS complex by 0.04 second.

B. Measure the intervals between two consecutive R waves in the QRS complexes. Then compare R-R intervals in several cycles.

C. Count the number of P waves and multiply by 10.

D. Multiply the number of small squares between the start of the QRS complex and the end of the T wave and multiply by 0.04 second.

■ You make the call

Describe in detail the two different methods used in these illustrations to determine atrial or ventricular rhythm.

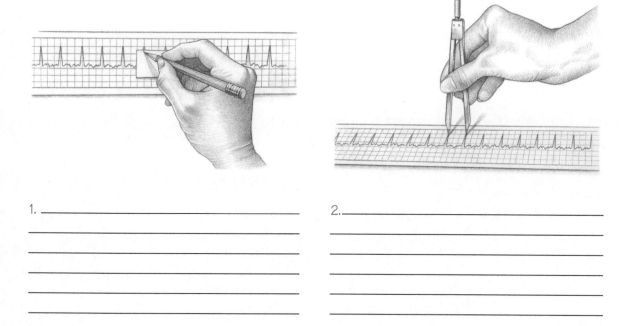

1. _____
_____
_____
_____
_____

2. _____
_____
_____
_____
_____

■ You make the call

Using the space provided, describe the characteristics of this rhythm strip.

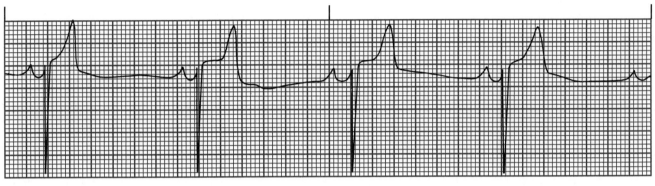

Atrial rhythm: _____

Ventricular rhythm: _____

Atrial rate: _____

Ventricular rate: _____

P wave: _____

PR interval: _____

QRS complex: _____

T wave: _____

QT interval: _____

Other: _____

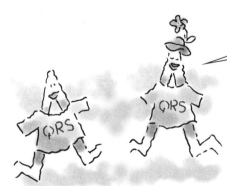

Where have you been? I've been waiting 0.18 second. Don't tell me there was another ventricular conduction delay.

■■
■ Boxing match

Fill in the answers to the clues below by using all of the syllables in the box. The number of syllables for each answer is shown in parentheses. Use each syllable only once. The first answer has been provided for you as an example.

AL	ATRI	BASE	COV	ERY	IR
PEAK	LAR	LAR	LINE	QUENCE	RE
REG	RHYTHM	SE	TRIC	U	U	VEN

1. Relating to or affecting an atrium   (2) A T R I A L

2. A set of observations or data used for comparison   (2) _ _ _ _ _ _ _

3. The maximum point   (1) _ _ _ _

4. Relating to a ventricle   (4) _ _ _ _ _ _ _ _ _ _

5. Regaining or returning to a normal state   (3) _ _ _ _ _ _ _

6. The pattern of recurrence of the cardiac cycle   (1) _ _ _ _ _ _

7. Failing to occur at regular intervals   (4) _ _ _ _ _ _ _ _ _

8. A continuous or connected series   (2) _ _ _ _ _ _ _ _

■■
■ Hit or miss

Some of the following statements are true; the others are false. Label each one accordingly.

_____ 1. Atrial and ventricular rates fall between 60 and 100 bpm for a normal sinus rhythm.

_____ 2. The sequence method uses the following numbers to establish heart rate: 300, 150, 100, 75, 50, and 25.

_____ 3. Measure the distance between R-R intervals to determine the atrial rhythm.

_____ 4. The QRS complex has no horizontal components.

> **Pep talk**
>
> " Those who would attain to any marked degree of excellence in a chosen pursuit must work, and work hard for it, prince or peasant. "
>
> —Bayard Taylor

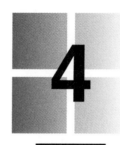

4

Sinus node arrhythmias

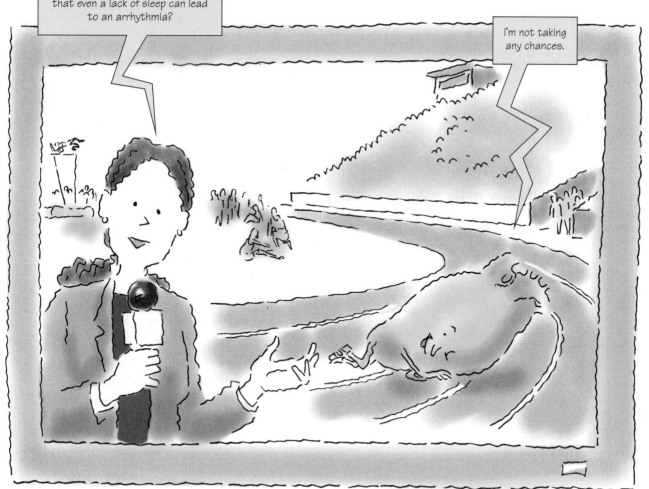

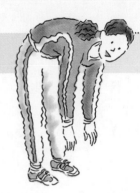

Warm-up

Sinus node arrhythmias review

Sinoatrial node

- Acts as primary pacemaker
- Inherent firing rate of 60 to 100 times/minute in a resting adult
- Supplied by blood from the right coronary artery and left circumflex artery

Sinus arrhythmia

Characteristics

- *Rhythms:* Irregular, corresponding to the respiratory cycle
- *Rates:* Within normal limits; vary with respiration
- *Other parameters:* QT interval variations

Treatment

- No treatment if patient is asymptomatic
- Correction of the underlying cause

Sinus bradycardia

Characteristics

- *Rhythms:* Regular
- *Rates:* Less than 60 beats/minute
- *Other parameters:* Normal

Treatment

- No treatment if patient is asymptomatic
- Correction of the underlying cause
- Temporary pacing to increase heart rate
- Atropine or epinephrine to maintain heart rate
- Dopamine for hypotension
- Permanent pacing if necessary

Sinus tachycardia

Characteristics

- *Rhythms:* Regular
- *Rates:* Both equal, generally 100 to 160 beats/minute
- *PR interval:* Normal
- *QRS complex:* Normal
- *T wave:* Normal
- *QT interval:* Shortened

Treatment

- No treatment if patient is asymptomatic
- Correction of the underlying cause
- Beta-adrenergic blockers or calcium channel blockers if symptomatic

Sinus arrest

Characteristics

- *Rhythms:* Regular, except for missing PQRST complex
- *Rates:* Equal and usually within normal limits; may vary as a result of pauses
- *P wave:* Normal and constant when present; absent during pause
- *QRS complex:* Normal when present; absent during pause
- *T wave:* Normal when present; absent during pause
- *QT interval:* Normal when present; absent during pause

Treatment

- No treatment if patient is asymptomatic
- Correction of the underlying cause
- Atropine or epinephrine to maintain heart rate
- Temporary pacemaker to maintain adequate cardiac output and perfusion
- Permanent pacemaker if necessary

Sick sinus syndrome

Characteristics

- *Rhythms:* Irregular with sinus pauses and abrupt rate changes
- *Rates:* Fast, slow, or combination of both
- *P wave:* Variations with rhythm and usually before QRS complex
- *QRS complex:* Normal
- *T wave:* Normal
- *QT interval:* Normal; variations with rhythm changes

Treatment

- No treatment if patient is asymptomatic
- Correction of the underlying cause
- Atropine or epinephrine for symptom-producing brady-cardia
- Temporary or permanent pacemaker if necessary
- Antiarrhythmics, such as metoprolol and digoxin, for tachy-arrhythmias
- Anticoagulants if atrial fibrillation develops

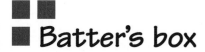

■ Batter's box

Before we really start to sweat, let's see if you've got your arrhythmias game on. Fill in the blanks below with the correct answer. *Hint:* Some answers are used more than once.

> It will take practice to master some of these arrhythmia concepts.

Arrhythmia essentials

When the heart functions normally, the sinoatrial (SA) node, acts as the primary

_____ . The sinus node assumes this role because its automatic
    1

_____ exceeds that of the heart's other pacemakers. In an adult at rest, the
    2

sinus node has an inherent firing rate of _____ to _____
                                                3   4

times/minute.

    The SA node's blood supply comes from the right _____ artery or the left
                                                                    5

_____ artery. The _____ nervous system innervates the sinus
    6   7

node through the _____ nerve, a _____ nerve, and several
                        8   9

_____ nerves. Stimulation of the _____ nerve decreases the
    10   11

node's firing rate, and stimulation of the _____ increases it.
                                                  12

Out of sync

In sinus _____ , the pacemaker cells of the _____ fire
              13   14

irregularly. Sinus _____ is characterized by a sinus rate below
                        15

_____ beats/minute and a _____ rhythm, whereas sinus
    16   17

_____ in an adult is characterized by a sinus rate of more than
    18

_____ beats/minute. A disorder of impulse formation, sinus
    19

_____ is caused by a lack of electrical activity in the _____ ,
    20   21

a condition also called _____ .
                              22

Options

60

100

Arrest

Arrhythmia

Atrial standstill

Atrium

Autonomic

Bradycardia

Circumflex

Coronary

Firing rate

Pacemaker

Parasympathetic

Regular

SA node

Sympathetic

Sympathetic system

Tachycardia

Vagus

■ Hit or miss

Some of the following statements are true; the others are false. Label each one accordingly.

_____ 1. During expiration, an increase in the flow of blood back to the heart increases the heart rate.

_____ 2. Sinus arrhythmia usually isn't significant and produces no symptoms.

_____ 3. In sinus arrhythmia, the cardiac rate stays within normal limits, but the rhythm is irregular.

_____ 4. Sinus arrhythmia is easier to detect when the heart rate is fast.

_____ 5. If sinus arrhythmia is unrelated to respirations, treatment may be necessary.

■ Jumble gym

Use the clues to help you unscramble words related to sinus arrhythmias. Then use the circled letters to form a word that correctly answers the question below.

Question: The doctor should be notified immediately if a sinus arrhythmia develops after a patient has taken what drug?

1. Sinus arrhythmia results from an inhibition of what?

   L G V A A O E N T __ __ ◯ __ __   __ ◯ __ __

2. Venous blood flow to the heart decreases during which respiratory phase?

   A I X P N E I R T O __ ◯ __ __ __ __ __ __ __ __

3. Cardiac conduction typically begins where?

   U S I S N E O D N __ ◯ __ __ __   __ __ ◯ __

4. Sinus arrhythmia corresponds with what physical activity?

   R A N E T I P S I R O __ __ __ __ ◯ __ __ __ __ __ ◯

Answer: __ __ __ __ __ __ __

Coaching session
Avoid a miscall

It isn't difficult to mistake a sinus arrhythmia for other rhythms. At first glance, it may look like atrial fibrillation, normal sinus rhythm with premature atrial contractions, SA block, or sinus pauses. To make the correct determination, observe the monitor and the patient's respiratory pattern for several minutes. And, as always, check the patient's pulse.

You make the call

Interpret this rhythm strip by first describing the distinguishing characteristics and then identifying the arrhythmia.

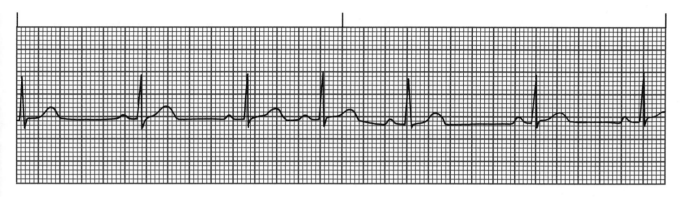

Rhythm: _____

Rate: _____

P wave: _____

PR interval: _____

QRS complex: _____

T wave: _____

QT interval: _____

Other: _____

Arrhythmia: _____

> As an athlete, I keep my heart in tip-top shape, so sinus bradycardia is run-of-the-mill for me.

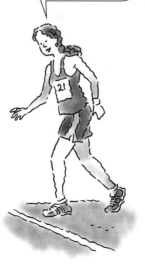

Strike out

Some of the statements below about sinus bradycardia are incorrect.
Cross out the incorrect statements.

1. In sinus bradycardia, vagal stimulation decreases and sympathetic stimulation increases.

2. Even if a patient is asymptomatic, sinus bradycardia is a serious condition that requires treatment.

3. For some patients, the signs and symptoms of sinus bradycardia include hypotension and dizziness.

4. In sinus bradycardia, the atrial and ventricular rhythms and rates are regular, except that they're both under 60 beats/minute.

■ Starting lineup

Put the following steps for treating sinus bradycardia in the correct order.

Administer dopamine, 5 to 20 mcg/kg/minute; administer epinephrine 2 to 10 mcg/minute.

Start an I.V. line, attach a monitor, and give I.V. fluids.

Obtain and review a 12-lead ECG.

Perform transcutaneous pacing, if available.

Administer atropine, 0.5 to 1 mg. Repeat doses every 3 to 5 minutes to a total of 0.04 mg/kg.

1.

2.

3.

4.

5.

■ Fair or foul?

Can you identify the causes of sinus bradycardia? Circle the causes that are correct.

1. Certain drugs, especially beta-adrenergic blockers, digoxin, and antiarrhythmics

2. Conditions producing excess vagal stimulation or decreased sympathetic stimulation

3. Compensatory mechanism in shock or anemia

4. Noncardiac disorders, such as hyperkalemia, increased intracranial pressure, and glaucoma

5. Response to stress, emotion, or fear

■ Match point

Match each term on the left with the correct explanation on the right.

1. Stokes-Adams attack _____
2. Acute inferior wall MI _____
3. Epinephrine _____
4. Dopamine _____

A. This drug should be administered if low blood pressure accompanies bradycardia.

B. Sinus bradycardia is considered a good prognostic sign in patients with this type of heart damage.

C. This disorder causes a sudden episode of light-headedness or loss of consciousness as a result of abrupt slowing or stopping of the heartbeat.

D. If atropine is ineffective in the treatment of bradycardia, this drug should be administered at a rate of 2 to 10 mcg/minute.

■ Hit or miss

Some of the following statements about sinus tachycardia are true; the others are false. Label each one accordingly.

_____ 1. Among other things, sinus tachycardia may be caused by exercise, hypovolemia, hemorrhage, or pain.

_____ 2. One cause of sinus tachycardia is acute inferior wall myocardial infarction.

_____ 3. Sinus tachycardia may be associated with massive heart damage, heart failure, or cardiogenic shock.

_____ 4. In tachycardia, decreased ventricular volume leads to hypotension and decreased peripheral perfusion.

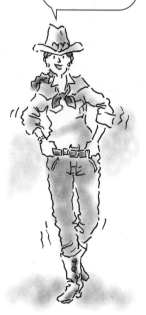

You've got a flair for sinus arrhythmias! Keep the rhythm going.

■ ■
■ **You make the call**

Interpret this rhythm strip by first describing the distinguishing characteristics and then identifying the arrhythmia.

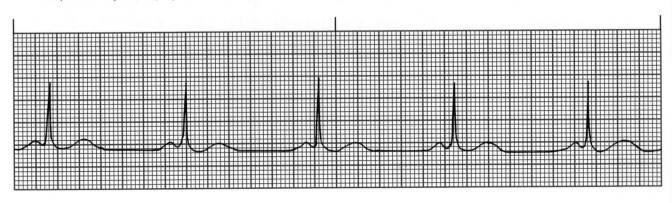

Rhythm: _____

Rate: _____

P wave: _____

PR interval: _____

QRS complex: _____

T wave: _____

QT interval: _____

Other: _____

Arrhythmia: _____

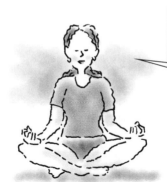

If you want to reduce your chances of tachycardia, take control. Focus on having a calm, relaxed mind. Crossword puzzles can be very relaxing, too.

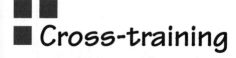

Cross-training

Complete this crossword puzzle using the clues below.

Across

2. In sinus tachycardia, the P wave may increase in _____

4. A symptom of heart failure

7. A beta-adrenergic blocker used to treat tachycardia

8. A common cause of tachycardia that doesn't produce symptoms

Down

1. Tachycardia worsens myocardial _____ by increasing the heart's demand for oxygen and reducing the duration of diastole

3. Normally, ventricular volume reaches 120 to 130 ml during _____

5. In sinus tachycardia, atrial and ventricular rhythms are _____

6. The "L" in LOC

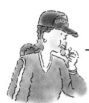

Coaching session

What happens in tachycardia

Tachycardia can lower cardiac output because it reduces ventricular filling time and the amount of blood that the ventricles pump during each contraction. Decreased ventricular volume leads to hypotension and decreased peripheral perfusion. As cardiac output drops, arterial pressure and peripheral perfusion decrease, worsening myocardial ischemia.

You make the call

Interpret this rhythm strip by first describing the distinguishing characteristics and then identifying the arrhythmia.

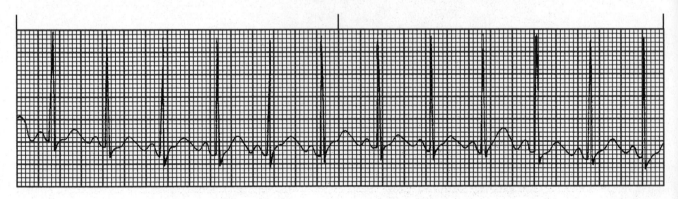

Rhythm: _____

Rate: _____

P wave: _____

PR interval: _____

QRS complex: _____

T wave: _____

QT interval: _____

Other: _____

Arrhythmia: _____

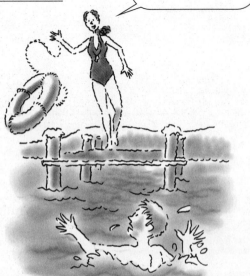

All of us need a little help at first, but keep at it, and you'll do swimmingly!

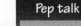

Pep talk

It does not matter how slowly you go so long as you do not stop.

—Confucius

▪ Strike out

Some of the statements below about sinus arrest are incorrect. Cross out the incorrect statements.

1. Atrial standstill is called *sinus arrest* when one or two beats aren't formed.

2. With sinus arrest, the length of the pause is a multiple of the previous R-R intervals.

3. A patient with sinus arrest may not feel the arrhythmias.

4. Activities that increase vagal stimulation increase the likelihood of sinus pauses.

▪ Power stretch

Stretch your knowledge of sinoatrial blocks by matching each of the arrhythmias listed here with its characteristics, listed on the right. Next, apply that knowledge by labeling the rhythm strip representative of each arrhythmia.

1. Second-degree type I block _____

2. Second-degree type II block _____

3. Third-degree block _____

A. Conduction time between the sinus node and the atrial tissue is normal until an impulse is blocked.

B. Conduction time between the sinus node and the surrounding atrial tissue becomes progressively longer until an entire cycle is dropped.

C. Some impulses are blocked, causing long sinus pauses.

D. The duration of the pause is less than twice the shortest P-P interval.

E. The duration of the pause is a multiple of the P-P interval.

F. The pause isn't a multiple of the sinus rhythm.

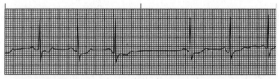

Rhythm strip 1 _____

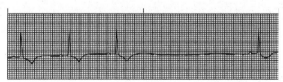

Rhythm strip 2 _____

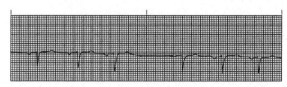

Rhythm strip 3 _____

▪▪ You make the call

Interpret this rhythm strip by first describing the distinguishing characteristics and then identifying the arrhythmia.

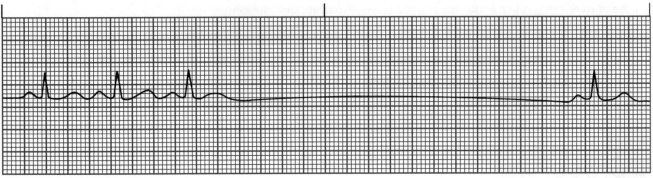

Rhythm: _____

Rate: _____

P wave: _____

PR interval: _____

QRS complex: _____

T wave: _____

QT interval: _____

Other: _____

Arrhythmia: _____

How's this for rhythm?

▪▪ Jumble gym

Unscramble these terms related to sinus arrest. Then use the circled letters to answer the question below.

Question: A patient with sinus arrest may exhibit what symptom?

1. USSNI SAUEP   _ _ ◯ _ _   _ _ _ ◯ _

2. RHMRATYIHA   _ _ _ _ ◯ _ _ _ _ _

3. IRDCCAA UTOTPU   ◯ _ _ _ _ _ _   ◯ _ _ _ _ _

4. CKRAMEPAE   ◯ _ _ ◯ _ _ _ _ _

Answer: _ _ _ _ _ _ _ _

■ Match point

See if you can match the terms relating to sick sinus syndrome on the left with the correct explanation on the right.

1. Metoprolol _____

2. Bradycardia-tachycardia syndrome _____

3. Anticoagulants _____

4. Blurred vision _____

A. Helps prevent thromboembolism and stroke

B. A term for a form of sick sinus syndrome

C. A symptom of decreased cardiac output

D. Used to treat tachyarrhythmias

■ Cross-training

Answer these questions to complete this crossword puzzle and text your knowledge of sinus node arrhythmias.

Across

2. Rhythm exhibited in sick sinus syndrome

4. A cause of trauma to the SA node

6. Potential result of thromboembolism

8. Sick sinus syndrome is also known as sinus nodal _____

11. Sinus arrest occurs when _____ or more beats aren't formed

Down

1. In sick sinus syndrome, the P wave _____ with the rhythm

3. When caring for a patient with sick sinus syndrome, a nurse should be alert for signs and symptoms of an _____

4. Atrial standstill is called sinus _____ when one or two beats aren't formed

5. A determining factor in the significance of sick sinus syndrome

7. This may be fast, slow, or normal in a patient with sick sinus syndrome

9. A patient with sinus arrest may develop this symptom

10. Sinus arrest is also called _____ block

■ You make the call

Interpret this rhythm strip by first describing the distinguishing characteristics and then identifying the arrhythmia.

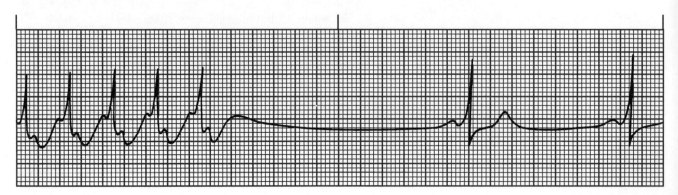

Rhythm: _____

Rate: _____

P wave: _____

PR interval: _____

QRS complex: _____

T wave: _____

QT interval: _____

Other: _____

Arrhythmia: _____

> Way to go!
> You've made great
> strides toward
> understanding
> sinus arrhythmias.

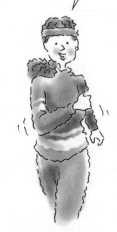

■ Train your brain

Sound out each group of pictures and symbols to reveal a statement about sinoatrial block.

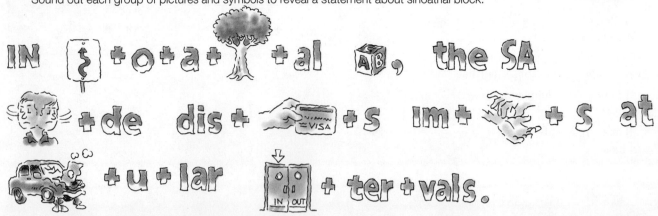

5

Atrial arrhythmias

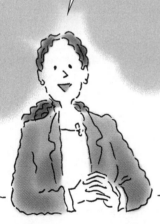

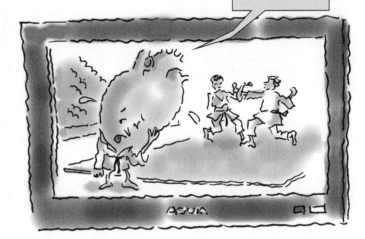

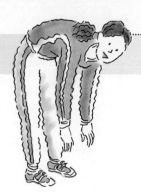

Atrial arrhythmias review

Premature atrial contractions

Characteristics

■ *Rhythms:* Irregular as a result of PACs
■ *P wave:* Premature with an abnormal configuration; may be buried in the previous T wave
■ *PR interval:* Usually normal; may be slightly shortened or prolonged
■ *QRS complex:* Similar to the underlying QRS complex when PAC is conducted; may not follow the premature P wave when a nonconducted PAC occurs

Treatment

■ No treatment if patient is asymptomatic
■ Correction of the underlying cause
■ Drugs, such as digoxin, procainamide, and quinidine, to prolong the atrial refractory period

Atrial tachycardia

Characteristics

■ *Rhythms:* Atrial—regular, irregular in multifocal atrial tachycardia (MAT); ventricular—regular when the block is constant and irregular when it isn't
■ *Rates:* Atrial—three or more successive ectopic atrial beats at a rate of 140 to 250 beats/minute; ventricular—varies
■ *P wave:* A 1:1 ratio with QRS complex (unless a block is present); may not be discernible; may be hidden in previous ST segment or T wave; in MAT, at least three different P waves seen
■ *PR interval:* Sometimes not measurable; varies in MAT
■ *QRS complex:* Usually normal
■ *T wave:* Normal or inverted
■ *QT interval:* Usually within normal limits; may be shorter
■ *ST-segment and T-wave changes:* Sometimes with ischemia

Treatment

■ Correction of underlying cause
■ Monitoring of blood digoxin levels for toxicity
■ Valsalva's maneuver or carotid sinus massage
■ Calcium channel blocker, beta-adrenergic blocker, or digoxin; synchronized cardioversion
■ Atrial overdrive pacing to stop arrhythmia

Atrial flutter

Characteristics

■ *Rhythms:* Atrial—regular; ventricular—depends on the atrioventricular (AV) conduction pattern
■ *Rates:* Atrial usually greater than ventricular
■ *P waves:* Abnormal with saw-toothed appearance
■ *QRS complex:* Usually normal; may be widened if waves are buried in complex
■ *T wave:* Unidentifiable
■ *QT interval:* Unmeasurable

Treatment

■ Anticoagulation therapy before converting rhythm if flutter is present for more than 48 hours
■ Digoxin, diltiazem, or amiodarone to control rate if heart function is impaired; synchronized cardioversion or amiodarone to convert rhythm if less than 48 hours

Atrial fibrillation

Characteristics

■ *Rhythms:* Irregularly irregular
■ *Rates:* Atrial—usually greater than 400 beats/minute; ventricular—varies from 100 to 150 beats/minute but can be lower
■ *P waves:* Absent
■ *f waves:* Seen as uneven baseline on ECG rather than distinguishable P waves
■ *R-R intervals:* Wide variation

Treatment

■ Anticoagulation therapy before converting rhythm if flutter is present for more than 48 hours
■ Digoxin, diltiazem, or amiodarone to control rate if heart function is impaired; synchronized cardioversion or amiodarone to convert rhythm if less than 48 hours

■ Cross-training

Complete the crossword using the clues below.

Across

2. A cause of asymptomatic PACs

4. Blocked PACs don't trigger this complex

5. The chief way to differentiate between nonconducted PACs and type II second-degree AV block is that, in type II second-degree AV block, the P-P interval is

   _____

9. In a patient with acute MI, PACs can serve as an early sign of a _____ imbalance

10. PACs originate _____ the SA node

12. The ability of cardiac cells to initiate impulses on their own

13. PACs occurring every other beat

Down

1. The hallmark ECG characteristic of a PAC is a _____ P wave

3. The A in PAC

6. Impulses driving atrial tachycardia originate _____ the ventricles

7. Commonly follows a PAC

8. Neurohormone released during pain or anxiety

11. The _____ of an ectopic focus determines whether the PR interval is normal, shortened, or slightly prolonged

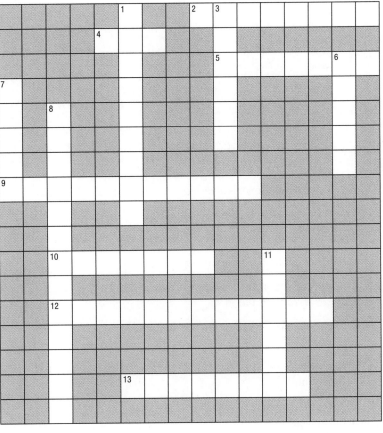

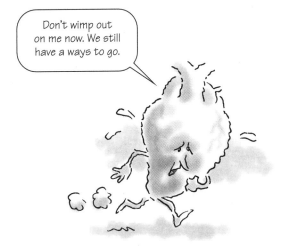

Don't wimp out on me now. We still have a ways to go.

■ Boxing match

Pull on your gloves and fill in the answers to these clues by using all of the syllables in the boxes. The number of syllables for each answer is shown in parentheses. Don't pull any punches—use each syllable only once. The first answer has been provided for you to help you get started.

AL	AL	ATRI	ATRI	AU	CAR	CON
DIA	DUC	EC	EN	ER	I	IC
~~IM~~	IZA	KICK	LAR	MA	MAK	NO
PACE	PO	~~PULSE~~	RE	RE	SI	TACHY
TIC	TION	TION	TO	TOP	TRY	TY

1. A wave of excitation transmitted through tissues — (2) I M P U L S E

2. The node that depolarizes early in PACs — (4) _ _ _ _ _ _ _ _ _

3. Delayed impulse in a one-way conduction path — (3) _ _ _ _ _ _ _

4. Occurring in an abnormal position — (3) _ _ _ _ _ _

5. Contraction that provides the ventricles with 15% to 25% of their blood — (3) _ _ _ _ _ _ _ _ _ _

6. Ability of a cardiac cell to initiate an impulse on its own — (6) _ _ _ _ _ _ _ _ _ _ _ _

7. Transmission of electrical impulses through the myocardium — (3) _ _ _ _ _ _ _ _ _

8. Group of cells that generates impulses to the heart muscle — (3) _ _ _ _ _ _ _

9. Recovery of the myocardial cells after depolarization — (5) _ _ _ _ _ _ _ _ _ _ _ _ _

10. Relatively rapid heart action — (3) _ _ _ _ _ _ _ _ _ _

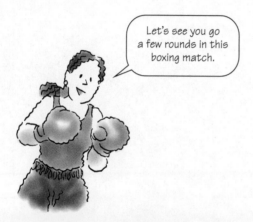

Let's see you go a few rounds in this boxing match.

You make the call

Interpret this rhythm strip by first describing the distinguishing characteristics and then identifying the arrhythmia.

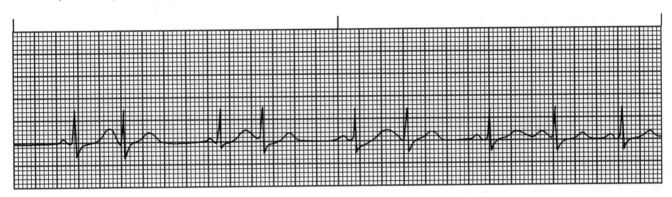

Rhythm: _____

Rate: _____

P wave: _____

PR interval: _____

QRS complex: _____

T wave: _____

QT interval: _____

Other: _____

Arrhythmia: _____

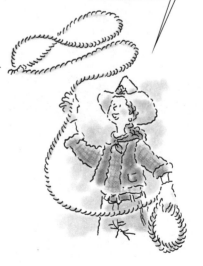

Howdy partner.
Here's your chance
to wrangle up some
facts on atrial
tachycardias.

■ Strike out

Some of the statements below about atrial tachycardia are incorrect. Cross out the incorrect statements.

1. Three or more successive ectopic atrial beats at a rate of 100 to 120 beats/minute characterize atrial tachycardia.

2. Atrial tachycardia is a supraventricular tachycardia.

3. Hyperthyroidism is the most common cause of atrial tachycardia.

4. A decrease in myocardial consumption and an increase in oxygen supply result from atrial tachycardia.

5. Atrial tachycardia is usually associated with primary or secondary cardiac problems.

■ Power stretch

Stretch your knowledge of atrial tachycardias by matching each of the arrhythmias listed here with its characteristics, listed to the right. Next, apply that knowledge by labeling the rhythm strip representative of each arrhythmia.

1. Atrial tachycardia with 2:1 block _____

2. Multifocal atrial tachycardia _____

3. Paroxysmal atrial tachycardia _____

A. Exhibits brief periods of tachycardia alternating with normal sinus rhythm

B. Has an irregular atrial and ventricular rhythm

C. Starts and stops suddenly

D. Contains two P waves for every QRS

E. Has a regular atrial rhythm; ventricular rhythm may be regular or irregular

F. Occurs when numerous atrial foci fire intermittently

G. Caused by increased automaticity of atrial tissue

H. Exhibits at least three different P-wave shapes

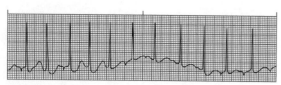

Rhythm strip 1 _____

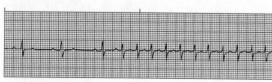

Rhythm strip 2 _____

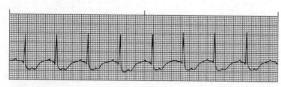

Rhythm strip 3 _____

You make the call

Interpret this rhythm strip by first describing the distinguishing characteristics and then identifying the arrhythmia.

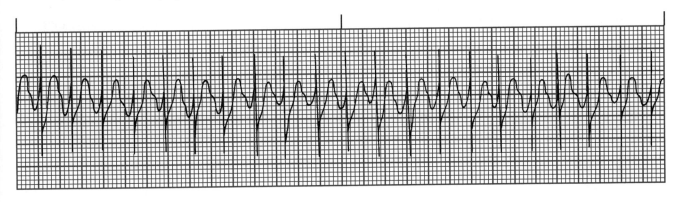

Rhythm: _____

Rate: _____

P wave: _____

PR interval: _____

QRS complex: _____

T wave: _____

QT interval: _____

Other: _____

Arrhythmia: _____

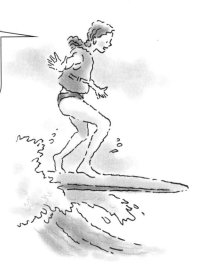

These waves are irregularly irregular. They looked saw-toothed at first, but now I see they're just erratic.

Pep talk

"Don't bunt. Aim out of the ballpark."
—David Ogilvy

■■ Fair or foul?

Can you identify the signs of digoxin toxicity? Circle the symptoms that are correct.

1. Hypotension

2. Cool, clammy skin

3. Confusion

4. Yellow-green halos around visual images

5. Hallucinations

6. Vomiting

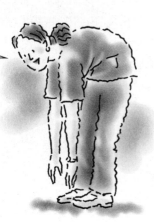

■■ You make the call

Using the space provided, explain what the nurse is doing in this illustration and why.

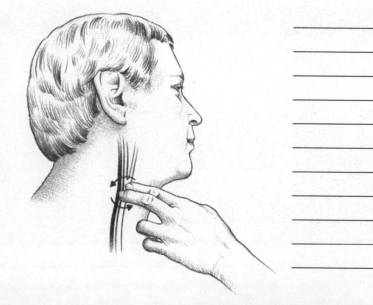

_____

_____

_____

_____

_____

_____

_____

_____

_____

_____

■ Hit or miss

Some of the following statements about atrial arrhythmias are true; the others are false. Label each one accordingly.

_____ 1. Rhythm strips for atrial tachycardia will show the ventricular rhythm is irregular when the block is constant and regular when it isn't.

_____ 2. A patient with MAT may complain about a sudden fast heartbeat or palpitations.

_____ 3. An atrial tachycardia is diagnosed by identifying P wave morphology on the 12-lead ECG.

_____ 4. Rhythms caused by increased automaticity don't respond to cardioversion.

_____ 5. Verapamil, beta-adrenergic blockers, and propafenone should only be used in patients with impaired left ventricular function.

■ Fair or foul?

The rhythm strip below illustrates atrial flutter. Circle the characteristics listed below that correctly describe this rhythm.

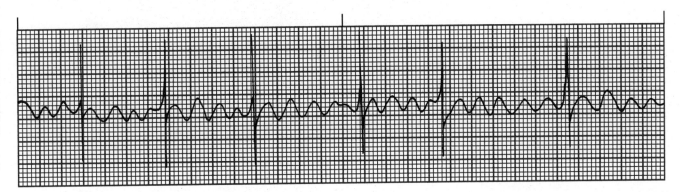

1. Rhythm: Atrial irregular; ventricular regular

2. Rate: Atrial 280 beats/minute; ventricular 60 beats/minute

3. P wave: Classic saw-toothed appearance

4. PR interval: Identical for each cycle

5. QRS complex: 0.08 second

6. T wave: Abnormal with some embedded P waves

7. QT interval: Unidentifiable

8. Other: None

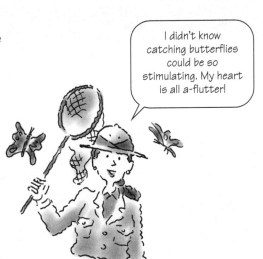

I didn't know catching butterflies could be so stimulating. My heart is all a-flutter!

■ Strike out

Some of the statements below about atrial flutter are incorrect. Cross out the incorrect statements.

1. Atrial flutter with rapid ventricular response and reduced cardiac output requires immediate intervention.

2. Synchronized cardioversion should never be used on a patient with atrial flutter.

3. Atrial flutter is characterized by abnormal T waves that produce a saw-toothed appearance.

4. Atrial flutter is commonly associated with second-degree block.

5. Atrial flutter usually results from an irritable spot, or focus, in the atria that takes over as pacemaker for one or more beats.

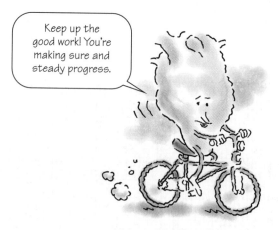

Keep up the good work! You're making sure and steady progress.

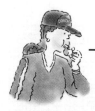

Coaching session
Atrial flutter or sinus tachycardia?

Whenever you see sinus tachycardia with a rate of 150 beats/minute, take another look. That rate is a common one for atrial flutter with 2:1 conduction. Look closely for flutter waves. They may be difficult to see if they're hidden in the QRS complex. You may need to check another lead to see them clearly.

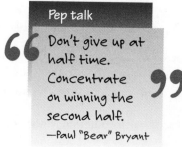

Pep talk

Don't give up at half time. Concentrate on winning the second half.

—Paul "Bear" Bryant

■ Jumble gym

Use the clues to help you unscramble words related to atrial flutter. Then use the circled letters to form a word that correctly answers the question.

Question: Atrial flutter may be caused by conditions that enlarge atrial tissue and elevate atrial what?

1. The faster the ventricular rate, the more dangerous the what?

   R M R A H I Y A T H _ Ⓞ _ _ _ _ _ _ _ _

2. Atrial flutter can possibly result from increased automaticity and what?

   E R E T N R Y _ Ⓞ _ _ _ Ⓞ _

3. P waves that blend together in a saw-toothed appearance are called what type of waves?

   T E R F L U T _ _ Ⓞ _ _ Ⓞ _

4. Rapid ventricular rate can cause what type of edema?

   L O M P A R U N Y Ⓞ _ _ _ _ _ _ _ _

5. Atrial flutter sometimes occurs in patients after cardiac what?

   G E R Y S U R Ⓞ _ _ _ _ _ _

6. Atrial flutter originates in what type of atrial focus?

   G E L S I N Ⓞ _ _ _ _ _

7. The patient's peripheral or apical what may be normal?

   S E P U L _ _ _ Ⓞ _

Answer: _ _ _ _ _ _ _ _ _

■■
■ Hit or miss

Some of the following statements about atrial fibrillation are true; the others are false. Label each one accordingly.

_____ 1. Catecholamine release during exercise may trigger atrial fibrillation.

_____ 2. Atrial kick isn't lost in atrial fibrillation..

_____ 3. A patient with mitral stenosis tolerates atrial fibrillation poorly and may develop shock or heart failure.

_____ 4. When the ventricular response rate is below 100, atrial fibrillation is considered controlled.

_____ 5. Synchronized cardioversion is similar to defibrillation except that cardioversion generally requires higher energy levels.

■■
■ Jumble gym

Use the clues to help you unscramble terms related to atrial arrhythmias. Then use the circled letters to form a word that correctly answers the question.

Question: If the f waves are pronounced, atrial fibrillation is called what?

1. A patient with atrial fibrillation is at increased risk for developing what disease?

    S M Y C S E T I   L M I E B O   _ _ Ⓞ _ _ _ _ _   Ⓞ _ _ _ _ _

2. What treatment of atrial fibrillation is most successful when used within 48 hours of the arrhythmia's development?

    R O S C V R D O A I E I N   Ⓞ _ _ _ _ _ _ _ _ _ _ _ _

3. What condition may cause atrial fibrillation?

    P X I Y H A O   _ _ _ _ _ _ Ⓞ

4. Atrial fibrillation may significantly affect what?

    C R I D C A A   T P T U O U   _ _ Ⓞ _ _ _ _   Ⓞ _ _ _ _ _

Answer: __ __ __ __ __ __

■■ ■ Cross-training

Test your knowledge of terms related to atrial arrhythmias by completing this crossword puzzle.

Across

2. Atrial fibrillation rhythm is _____ irregular

6. A _____ defibrillator may be used to convert an atrial arrhythmia.

8. Like other atrial arrhythmias, atrial fibrillation eliminates atrial _____

9. In atrial tachycardia, the P wave is almost always _____

11. The AV node acts as a _____ to block excessive impulses

Down

1. During atrial fibrillation, the ectopic impulses fire 400 to 600 times/minute, causing the atria to _____

3. In atrial tachycardia, the ventricular rhythm is _____ when the block is constant

4. Occurring in bursts

5. For a patient with atrial fibrillation, assess both the apical and this pulse rate

7. Causes T waves to be inverted

9. Atrial flutter commonly occurs when atrial pressures are _____

10. Atrial fibrillation is called _____ if the f waves aren't pronounced

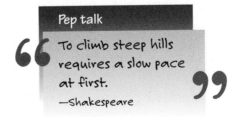

Pep talk

To climb steep hills requires a slow pace at first.
—Shakespeare

You make the call

Interpret this rhythm strip by first describing the distinguishing characteristics and then identifying the arrhythmia.

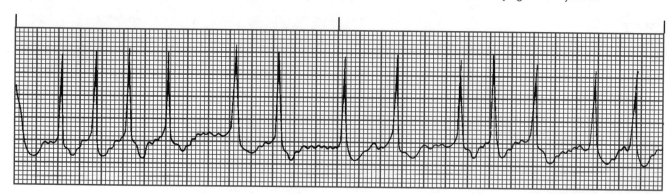

Rhythm: _____

Rate: _____

P wave: _____

PR interval: _____

QRS complex: _____

T wave: _____

QT interval: _____

Other: _____

Arrhythmia: _____

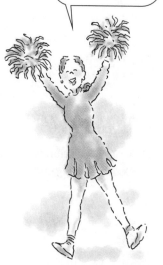

Give me an E!
Give me C!
Give me a G!
What are we going to comprehend?
E-C-Gs!

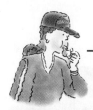

Coaching session
Synchronized cardioversion

A patient whose arrhythmia causes low cardiac output and hypotension may be a candidate for synchronized cardioversion. Synchronized cardioversion is similar to defibrillation except that cardioversion generally requires lower energy levels. The R wave on the patient's electrocardiogram is synchronized with the cardioverter (defibrillator). To stop atrial depolarization and reestablish normal sinus rhythm, stimulation must occur during the R wave. Be aware that synchronized cardioversion carries the risk of lethal arrhythmias when used in patients with digoxin toxicity.

Starting lineup

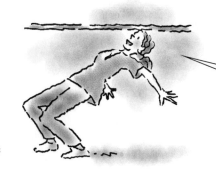

With your limber mind, I don't think you'll have to bend over backward to complete this next workout.

Put the following steps for treating a symptomatic patient with atrial fibrillation in the correct order.

Synchronize the defibrillator with the R wave on the patient's electrocardiogram.	1.
Administer anticoagulation therapy.	2.
Call, "All clear," and hold the paddles to the patient's chest until the energy is discharged.	3.
Administer moderate sedation.	4.
Place one paddle to the right of the upper sternum and one paddle over the fifth or sixth intercostal space at the left anterior axillary line.	5.

Train your brain

Sound out each group of pictures and symbols to discover an atrial arrhythmia precaution.

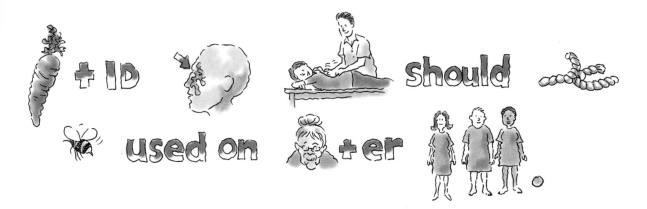

Power stretch

Stretch your knowledge of atrial arrhythmias by matching each of the arrhythmias listed here with its characteristics, listed on the right. Next, apply that knowledge by labeling the rhythm strip representative of each arrhythmia.

1. Atrial fibrillation _____

2. Atrial flutter _____

3. Normal sinus rhythm with PACs _____

A. Exhibits P waves with a classic saw-toothed appearance

B. Contains premature and abnormally shaped P waves

C. Most common arrhythmia

D. Commonly associated with second-degree block

E. Distinguished by the absence of P waves and an irregular ventricular response

F. May be mistaken as sinus tachycardia with a ventricular rate of 150

G. Has a regular baseline rhythm

H. Has an atrial rate that's almost indiscernible but is usually greater than 400 beats/minute

I. Has a regular atrial rate and an irregular ventricular rate

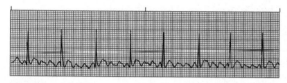

Rhythm strip 1 _____

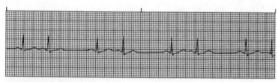

Rhythm strip 2 _____

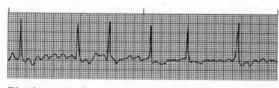

Rhythm strip 3 _____

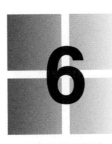

Junctional arrhythmias

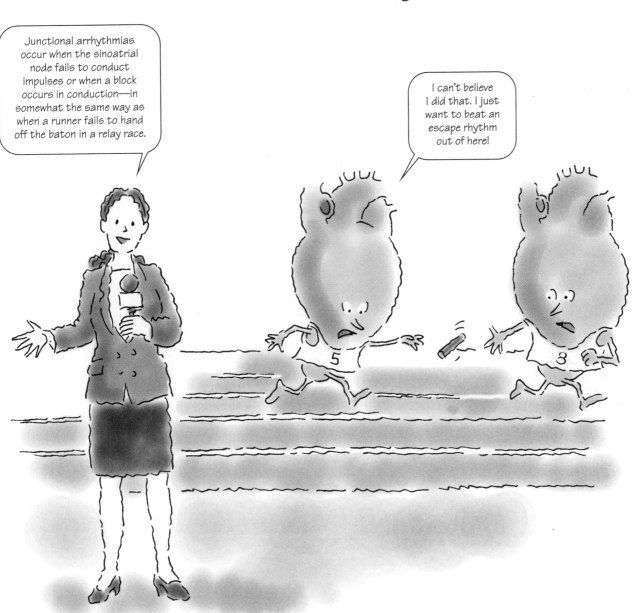

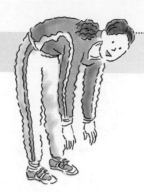

Junctional arrhythmias review

Overview of junctional arrhythmias

- Originate in the atrioventricular (AV) junction
- Occur when the sinoatrial (SA) node is suppressed or conduction is blocked
- Impulses cause retrograde depolarization and inverted P waves in leads II, III, and aV$_F$

Wolff-Parkinson-White syndrome

Characteristics

- *PR interval:* Less than 0.10 second
- *QRS complex:* Greater than 0.10 second; beginning of complex may have slurred appearance (delta wave)

Treatment

- No treatment if patient is asymptomatic
- Treatment of tachyarrhythmias as indicated
- Radiofrequency ablation if resistant to other treatments

Premature junctional contraction

Characteristics

- *Rhythms:* Irregular with PJC appearance
- *Rates:* Vary with underlying rhythm
- *P wave:* Inverted; occurs before, during, or after QRS complex; may be absent
- *PR interval:* Less than 0.12 second or unmeasurable
- *QRS complex:* Usually normal
- *T wave:* Usually normal
- *QT interval:* Usually normal
- *Other:* Sometimes a compensatory pause after PJC

Treatment

- No treatment if patient is asymptomatic
- Correction of the underlying cause
- Discontinuation of digoxin if indicated
- Reduction or elimination of caffeine intake

Junctional escape rhythm

Characteristics

- *Rhythms:* Regular
- *Rates:* 40 to 60 beats/minute
- *P wave:* Inverted in leads II, III, and aV$_F$; can occur before, during, or after QRS complex
- *PR interval:* Less than 0.12 second if P wave comes before QRS complex
- *QRS complex:* Normal; less than 0.12 second
- *T wave:* Normal
- *QT interval:* Normal

Treatment

- Correction of the underlying cause
- Atropine for symptom-producing bradycardia
- Temporary or permanent pacemaker insertion if arrhythmia refractory to drugs
- Discontinuation of digoxin if indicated

Accelerated junctional rhythm

Characteristics

- *Rhythms:* Regular
- *Rates:* 60 to 100 beats/minute
- *P wave:* Inverted in leads II, III, and aV$_F$ (if present); occurs before, during, or after QRS complex
- *PR interval:* Measurable only with P wave that comes before QRS complex; 0.12 second or less
- *QRS complex:* Normal
- *T wave:* Normal
- *QT interval:* Normal

Treatment

- Correction of the underlying cause
- Discontinuation of digoxin if indicated
- Temporary pacemaker insertion if patient is symptomatic

Junctional tachycardia

Characteristics

- *Rhythms:* Regular
- *Rates:* 100 to 200 beats/minute
- *P wave:* Inverted in leads II, III, aV$_F$; location varies around QRS complex
- *PR interval:* Shortened at less than 0.12 second or unmeasurable
- *QRS complex:* Normal
- *T wave:* Usually normal; may contain P wave
- *QT interval:* Usually normal

Treatment

- Correction of the underlying cause
- Discontinuation of digoxin if indicated
- Temporary or permanent pacemaker insertion if patient is symptomatic
- Vagal maneuvers or drugs such as verapamil to slow heart rate if patient is symptomatic

Wandering pacemaker

Characteristics

- *Rhythms:* Irregular
- *Rates:* Usually normal or below 60 beats/minute
- *P wave:* Changes in size and shape
- *PR interval:* Varies
- *QRS complex:* Usually normal
- *QT interval:* Sometimes varies

Treatment

- No treatment if patient is asymptomatic
- Correction of the underlying cause

Now, tie on your running shoes and see how fast you can get through this course on junctional arrhythmias.

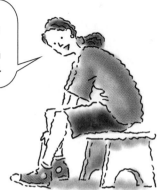

■ Batter's box

Fill in each blank with the correct answer. *Hint:* Some words are used more than once.

Junctional arrhythmia basics

Junctional arrhythmias originate in the _____ junction—the area
                                              1

around the _____ and the _____ . The arrhythmias
                    2   3

occur when the _____ , a higher _____ , is suppressed
                        4   5

and fails to conduct _____ or when a _____ occurs in
                              6   7

conduction. _____ impulses may then be initiated by pacemaker
                      8

_____ in the _____ .
         9   10

     In normal impulse conduction, the _____ slows transmission of
                                                        11

the _____ from the _____ to the _____ ,
          12   13   14

which gives the atria time to contract and _____ as much
                                                    15

_____ as they can into the ventricles before they contract.
        16

Impulses every which way

Because the AV junction is located in the _____ part of the
                                                    17

_____ near the _____ valve, _____
        18   19   20

generated in this area cause the heart to be _____ in an abnormal
                                                      21

way. The impulse moves _____ and causes backward, or
                                22

_____ , depolarization of the _____ and
        23   24

_____ P waves in leads _____ , _____ ,
        25   26   27

and _____ .
            28

Options

II

III

Atria

Atrioventricular

aV_F

AV junction

AV node

Block

Blood

Bundle of His

Cells

Depolarized

Electrical

Impulse

Impulses

Inverted

Lower

Pacemaker

Pump

Retrograde

Right atrium

Sinoatrial

Tricuspid

Upward

Ventricles

■■
■ Hit or miss

Some of the following statements are true; the others are false. Label each one accordingly.

_____ 1. Arrhythmias that cause inverted P waves on ECGs are always junctional in origin.

_____ 2. Wolff-Parkinson-White syndrome must be treated if tachyarrhythmias occur.

_____ 3. Junctional arrhythmias generate impulses so high in the atria that they cause antegrade depolarization of the atria.

_____ 4. To determine whether an arrhythmia is atrial or junction, look at the PR interval.

■■
■ Match point

Match each of the depolarization sequences on the left below with its appropriate rhythm strip.

1. Atria first _____

2. Ventricles first _____

3. Simultaneous _____

A.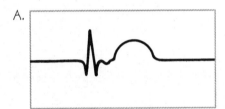

B.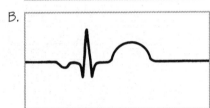

C.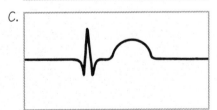

Coaching session
Wolff-Parkinson-White syndrome

In Wolff-Parkinson-White syndrome, conduction bypass develops outside the atrioventricular (AV) junction and connects the atria with the ventricles. It is typically a congenital rhythm disorder that occurs mainly in young children and in adults ages 20 to 35. This syndrome causes a shortened PR interval and a widened QRS complex. The beginning of the QRS complex may look slurred, forming the hallmark sign—known as a *delta wave*—of Wolff-Parkinson-White syndrome. This syndrome must be treated if tachyarrhythmias occur.

■■
■ Strike out

Some of the statements below are incorrect. Cross out the incorrect statements.

1. Atrial arrhythmias are sometimes mistaken for junctional arrhythmias.

2. An arrhythmia with a PR interval less than 0.12 second originated in the atria.

3. In normal impulse conduction, the SA node slows transmission of the impulse from the atria to the ventricles.

4. Wolff-Parkinson-White syndrome occurs mainly in older adults.

■■
■ You make the call

Interpret this rhythm strip by first describing the distinguishing characteristics and then identifying the arrhythmia.

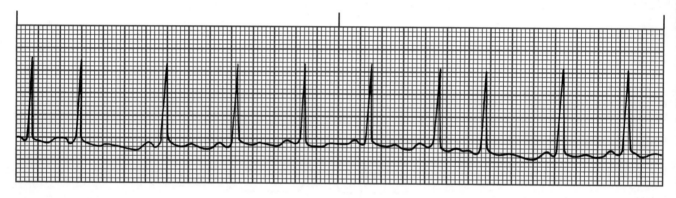

Rhythm: _____

Rate: _____

P wave: _____

PR interval: _____

QRS complex: _____

T wave: _____

QT interval: _____

Other: _____

Arrhythmia: _____

> This may look highly irregular, but what can I say? I just go with my impulses.

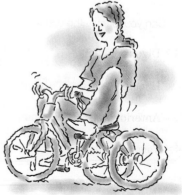

■ You make the call

Interpret this rhythm strip by first describing the distinguishing characteristics and then identifying the arrhythmia.

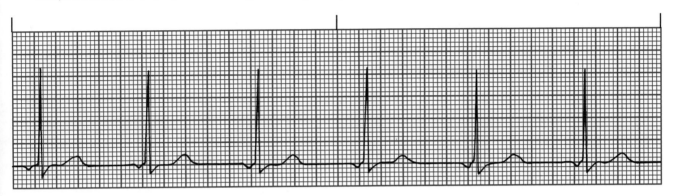

Rhythm: _____

Rate: _____

P wave: _____

PR interval: _____

QRS complex: _____

T wave: _____

QT interval: _____

Other: _____

Arrhythmia: _____

■ Fair or foul?

Can you identify the causes of junctional escape rhythm? Circle the causes that are correct.

1. Digoxin toxicity

2. Rheumatic heart disease

3. Anterior wall MI

4. Vagal stimulation

5. Advanced age

■ Jumble gym

Use the clues provided to help you unscramble words related to junctional arrhythmias. Then use the circled letters to form a word that correctly answers the question.

Question: What drug may be given to increase heart rate in a patient with a junctional escape rhythm?

1. May be used to treat junctional arrhythmias

   K E P A M C A R E ◯ _ _ _ _ _ _ ◯

2. Type of atrial conduction seen in junctional arrhythmias

   D R O R E G T R A E _ _ ◯ _ ◯ _ _ _ _ _

3. Mechanism that's enhanced in junctional escape rhythm

   I M O A Y T C A U T I T ◯ _ _ _ _ _ _ ◯ _ _ _ _

4. One possible symptom resulting from inadequate cardiac output

   P N E S C Y O _ _ ◯ _ _ _ ◯

Answer: __ __ __ __ __ __ __ __

■ Hit or miss

Some of the following statements about junctional rhythms are true; the others are false. Label each one accordingly.

_____ 1. A junctional rhythm is considered accelerated in infants and toddlers only when it's greater than 80 beats/minute.

_____ 2. One condition that can cause accelerated junctional arrhythmia is valvular heart disease.

_____ 3. With an accelerated junctional rhythm, look for an irregular rhythm.

_____ 4. Accelerated junctional rhythm has the same rate as sinus rhythm.

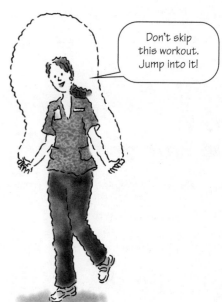

Don't skip this workout. Jump into it!

■ Cross-training

Complete the crossword puzzle using the clues below.

Across

2. Junctional rhythm in which an irritable focus in the AV junction speeds up to take over as the heart's pacemaker

6. A PJC appears as this type of beat on a rhythm strip

8. An impulse that moves upward causes this type of depolarization of the atria

10. A P wave falling during the QRS complex is

_____

11. Condition potentially caused by PJCs due to a transient decrease in cardiac output

Down

1. Patients with PJCs should be monitored for _____ instability

3. A PJC is a beat that occurs _____ a normal beat

4. The P in PJC

5. If ventricles depolarize first in a junctional rhythm, the P wave will appear _____ the QRS

7. Junctional escape beats may prevent ventricular

_____

9. PJCs may be caused by _____ levels greater than 2.5 ng/ml

■ Fair or foul?

The rhythm strip below depicts an accelerated junctional rhythm. Circle the distinguishing characteristics that are correct for this rhythm strip.

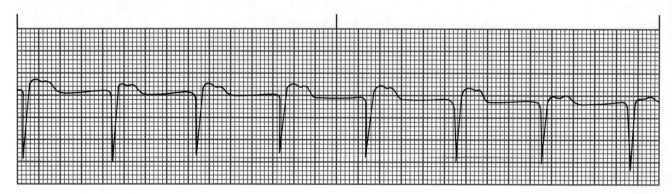

1. Rhythm: Regular

2. Rate: 100 beats/minute

3. P wave: Inverted and preceding each QRS complex

4. PR interval: Unmeasurable

5. QRS complex: 0.06 second

6. T wave: Unidentifiable

7. QT interval: 0.32 second

8. Other: None

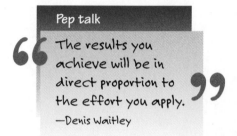

Pep talk

The results you achieve will be in direct proportion to the effort you apply.

—Denis Waitley

■ Match point

Match each of the terms on the left with its correct definition on the right.

1. Atrial flutter _____

2. Vagal maneuvers _____

3. Digoxin toxicity _____

4. Congenital heart disease _____

A. Most common cause of junctional tachycardias

B. Potential cause of junctional tachycardia in children

C. A type of supraventricular tachycardia

D. May slow the heart rate for symptomatic patients with junctional tachycardias

■ Strike out

Some of the statements below about junctional tachycardia are incorrect. Cross out the incorrect statements.

1. Two PJCs occur in a row in junctional tachycardia.

2. The rate is usually between 100 and 200 beats/minute.

3. A patient with recurrent junctional tachycardia may be treated with cardioversion.

4. If junctional tachycardia is a result of digoxin toxicity, the doctor may order digoxin immune fab.

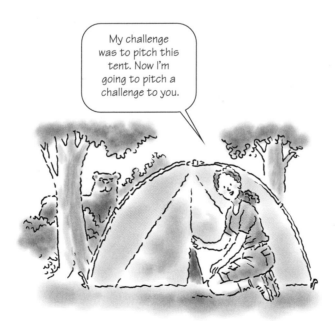

My challenge was to pitch this tent. Now I'm going to pitch a challenge to you.

You make the call

Interpret this rhythm strip by first describing the distinguishing characteristics and then identifying the arrhythmia.

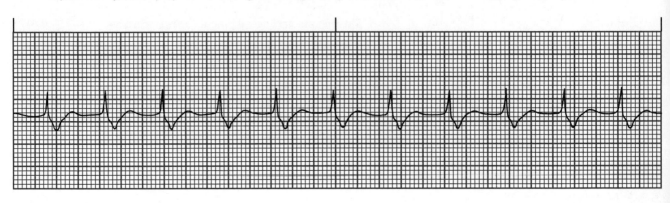

Rhythm: _____

Rate: _____

P wave: _____

PR interval: _____

QRS complex: _____

T wave: _____

QT interval: _____

Other: _____

Arrhythmia: _____

Cross-training

Complete the crossword puzzle to test your knowledge of junctional arrhythmias.

Across

1. Cause of wandering pacemaker: _____ carditis

3. Early beat with an inverted P wave and a PR interval less than 0.12 second

4. This attribute of wandering pacemaker arrhythmias makes them difficult to identify

8. Rhythm of wandering pacemaker on an ECG strip

10. Wandering pacemaker results from the heart's pacemaker changing its focus from the SA node to another area above the _____

Down

2. Patients with wandering pacemaker are generally unaware of the arrhythmia and are _____

5. In accelerated junctional rhythm, the QRS complex appears _____

6. Wandering pacemaker arrhythmias are common in _____

7. If the patient is symptomatic, mental _____ should be assessed

9. One place a wandering pacemaker impulse may originate

Match point

Match each type of arrhythmia on the left with its characteristics on the right.

1. Junctional escape rhythm _____

2. Accelerated junctional rhythm _____

3. Junctional tachycardia _____

4. Atrial arrhythmia _____

A. Has a regular rhythm with a rate between 60 and 100 beats/minute

B. Exhibits an inverted P wave before the QRS complex and a normal PR interval

C. Has a regular rhythm with a rate between 100 and 200 beats/minute

D. Exhibits a regular rhythm with a rate of 40 to 60 beats/minute

Fair or foul?

The rhythm strip below depicts a wandering pacemaker. Circle the distinguishing characteristics that are correct for this rhythm strip.

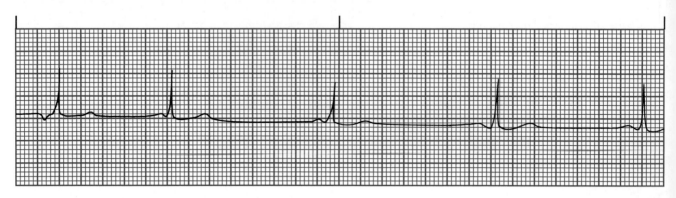

1. Rhythm: Irregular atrial and ventricular rhythms

2. Rate: Atrial and ventricular rates of 80 beats/minute

3. P wave: Changes in size and shape; first P wave inverted, second upright

4. PR interval: Variable

5. QRS complex: 0.10 second

6. T wave: Normal

7. QT interval: 0.32 second

8. Other: None

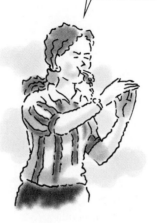

Time out! Foul on the Pacemakers for excessive wandering.

You make the call

Interpret this rhythm strip by first describing the distinguishing characteristics and then identifying the arrhythmia.

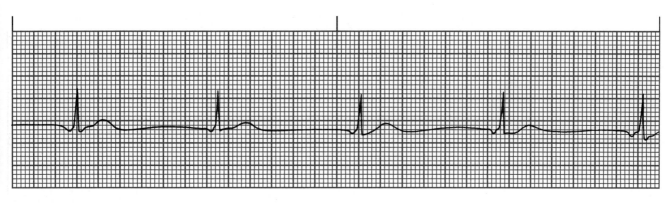

Rhythm: _____

Rate: _____

P wave: _____

PR interval: _____

QRS complex: _____

T wave: _____

QT interval: _____

Other: _____

Arrhythmia: _____

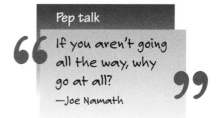

■ Power stretch

Stretch your knowledge of arrhythmias by first unscrambling the words on the left to reveal key terms. Then draw a line from each box to the correct explanation of each term.

BLANAIOT

— — — — — — —

DEGRANWIN MERKACAPE

— — — — — — — — —

— — — — — — — — —

DERVENTI

— — — — — — — —

NUCJTANIOL
THIAMHARYR

— — — — — — — — — —

— — — — — — — — — —

ATLED VEAW

— — — — — — — — —

TUNNJIOCAL
CHYATDRAAIC

— — — — — — — — — —

— — — — — — — — — — —

A. Negative or downward deflection on an ECG waveform

B. Arrhythmia originating in the atrioventricular junction

C. Irregular rhythm that results when the heart's pacemaker changes its focus from the SA node to another area above the ventricles

D. Surgical or radio-frequency removal of an irritable focus in the heart

E. Hallmark sign of Wolff-Parkinson-White syndrome

F. When three or more PJCs occur in a row

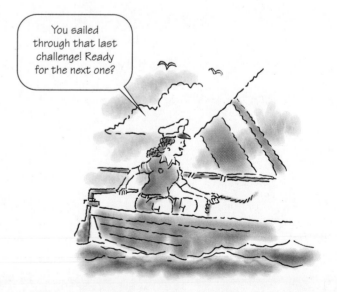

You sailed through that last challenge! Ready for the next one?

You make the call

Interpret this rhythm strip by first describing the distinguishing characteristics and then identifying the arrhythmia.

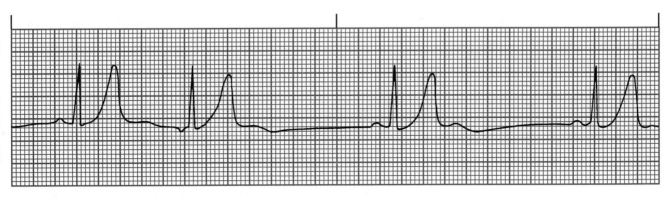

Rhythm: _____

Rate: _____

P wave: _____

PR interval: _____

QRS complex: _____

T wave: _____

QT interval: _____

Other: _____

Arrhythmia: _____

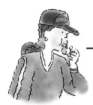

Coaching session
Junctional and supraventricular tachycardia

When a tachycardia has a narrow QRS complex, determining whether its source is junctional or atrial may be difficult. When the rate approaches 150 beats/minute, the P wave is hidden in the previous T wave, so you won't be able to use the P wave to decide where the rhythm originated. In such a case, call the rhythm *supraventricular* tachycardia, a general term that refers to the origin as being above the ventricles.

▇ Match point

Match each of the junctional arrhythmias on the left with its correct rhythm strip.

1. Junctional rhythm _____
2. Wandering pacemaker _____
3. Accelerated junctional rhythm _____

A.
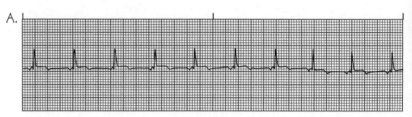

B.
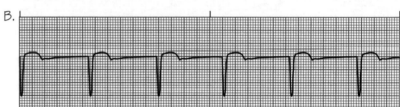

C.
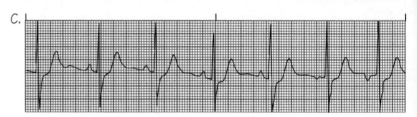

Now that you've finished this chapter, feel free to kick back and relax. You earned it. Then move on to the next chapter.

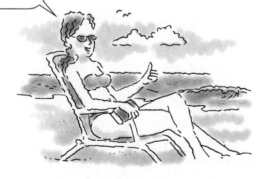

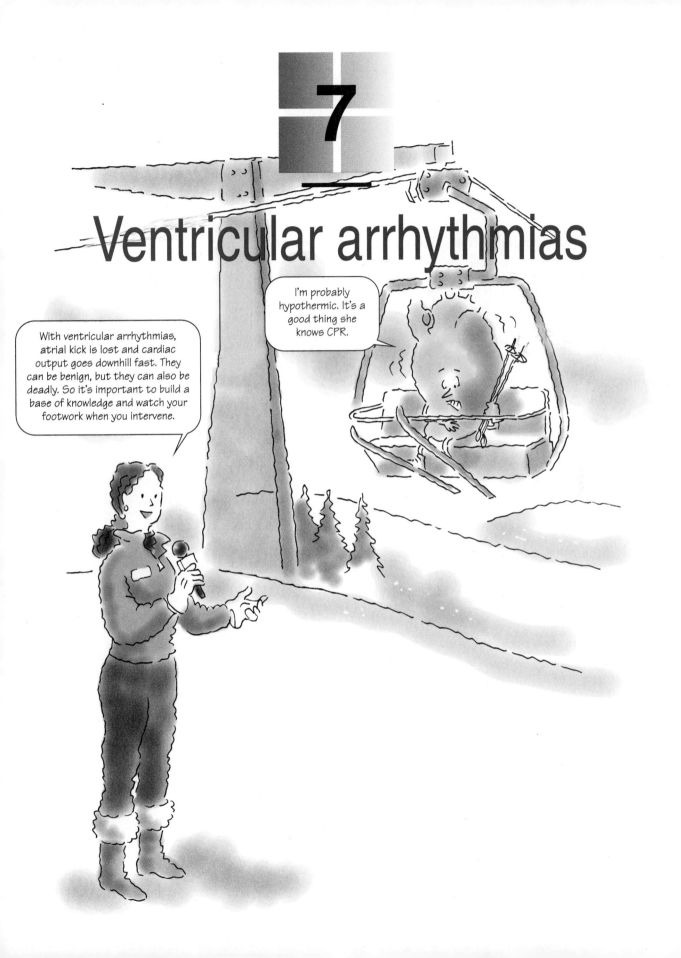

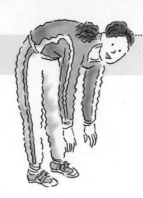

Warm-up

Ventricular arrhythmias review

Overview of ventricular arrhythmias

- Originate in the ventricles, below the bundle of His
- Loss of atrial kick, decreasing cardiac output
- Potentially fatal without treatment or resuscitation

Characteristics

- QRS complex wider than normal
- T wave and QRS complex deflect in opposite directions
- P wave is absent

Premature ventricular contraction

Characteristics

- *Rhythm:* Irregular during premature ventricular contraction (PVC); underlying rhythm may be regular
- *Rate:* Patterned after underlying rhythm
- *P wave:* Absent
- *PR interval:* Unmeasurable
- *QRS complex:* Wide and bizarre
- *T wave:* Opposite direction from QRS complex
- *QT interval:* Unmeasurable
- *Other:* Possible compensatory pause

Treatment

- Correction of the underlying cause
- Discontinuation of drug that may be causing toxicity
- Correction of electrolyte imbalances
- Procainamide, lidocaine, or amiodarone if warranted

Idioventricular rhythms

- Act as safety mechanism to prevent ventricular standstill
- Occur as escape beats, idioventricular rhythm, or accelerated idioventricular rhythm

Characteristics

- *Rhythm:* Atrial—undetermined; ventricular—usually regular
- *Rate:* Atrial—unmeasurable; ventricular—20 to 40 beats/minute
- *P wave:* Absent
- *PR interval:* Unmeasurable
- *QRS complex:* Wide and bizarre
- *T wave:* Deflection opposite that of QRS complex
- *QT interval:* Greater than 0.44 second

Treatment

- Atropine to increase heart rate
- Temporary or permanent pacemaker if arrhythmia is refractory to drugs
- Avoidance of drugs that suppress the idioventricular rhythm, such as lidocaine and other antiarrhythmics

Ventricular tachycardia

Characteristics

- *Rhythm:* Atrial—can't be determined; ventricular—regular or slightly irregular
- *Rate:* Atrial—can't be determined; ventricular—100 to 250 beats/minute
- *P wave:* Absent or hidden by QRS complex
- *PR interval:* Unmeasurable
- *QRS complex:* Wide and bizarre, with increased amplitude; duration greater than 0.12 second
- T wave: Opposite direction of QRS complex
- Other: Possible torsades de pointes

Treatment

Advanced cardiac life support (ACLS) protocols:
- Amiodarone; if patient is stable with monomorphic QRS complexes and drugs are unsuccessful, cardioversion
- Beta-adrenergic blockers, lidocaine, amiodarone, procainamide, or sotalol if patient's electrocardiogram (ECG) shows polymorphic QRS complexes and normal QT interval; cardioversion if unsuccessful
- Magnesium sulfate I.V. if patient shows polymorphic QRS and QT interval is prolonged, then overdrive pacing if rhythm persists (possibly also isoproterenol)
- Defibrillation; cardiopulmonary resuscitation (CPR), endotracheal intubation, and epinephrine or vasopressin, if patient is pulseless (possibly also consider amiodarone, lidocaine, or magnesium sulfate)
- Cardioverter-defibrillator possibly implanted for recurrent ventricular tachycardia

Torsades de pointes

- Form of polymorphic ventricular tachycardia
- Sometimes deteriorates into ventricular fibrillation

Characteristics

- *Rhythm:* Ventricular—irregular
- *Rate:* 150 to 250 beats/minute
- *P wave:* Usually absent
- *PR interval:* Unmeasurable
- *QRS complex:* Wide; rotates around the baseline; deflection downward and upward for several beats

Treatment

- Correction of the underlying cause
- Discontinuation of offending drug (usually one that lengthens the QT interval)
- Overdrive pacing
- Magnesium sulfate sometimes effective
- Cardioversion if unresponsive to other treatment

Ventricular fibrillation

- Electrical impulses arise from many different foci in the ventricles
- Produces no effective muscular contraction and no cardiac output
- If untreated, it causes most cases of sudden cardiac death out of hospital

Characteristics

- *Rhythm:* Can't be determined
- *Rate:* Can't be determined
- *P wave:* Can't be determined
- *PR interval:* Can't be determined
- *QRS complex:* Can't be determined
- *T wave:* Can't be determined
- *QT interval:* Isn't applicable
- *Other:* Variations in size of fibrillatory waves

Treatment

ACLS protocols:
- Defibrillation
- Initiation of CPR
- Endotracheal intubation and administration of epinephrine or vasopressin (consider amiodarone, lidocaine, magnesium sulfate, or procainamide)
- Implantation of cardioverter-defibrillator if patient is at risk for recurrent ventricular fibrillation

Asystole

- Characterized by ventricular standstill and cardiac arrest
- Fatal without prompt CPR and treatment

Characteristics

- Lack of electrical activity seen on ECG as a nearly flat line

Treatment

ACLS protocols:
- Initiation of CPR
- Endotracheal intubation, transcutaneous pacing, and epinephrine and atropine

Pulseless electrical activity

Characteristics

- Electrical activity is present on ECG but heart muscle can't contract
- Result is no palpable pulse or blood pressure and cardiac arrest

Treatment

ACLS protocols:
- Initiation of CPR
- Epinephrine
- Atropine for bradycardia
- Correction of the underlying cause

■ Batter's box

Before jumping into the workout, let's review a few key concepts. Fill in the blanks with the appropriate words. *Hint:* Words may be used more than once.

Ventricular arrhythmia essentials

Ventricular arrhythmias originate in the _____ below the

_____ . They occur when electrical impulses _____ the

_____ using a different pathway from normal impulses.

    Ventricular arrhythmias appear on an ECG in characteristic ways. The

_____ is wider than normal because of the prolonged conduction time

through the _____ . The _____ and the _____

deflect in _____ directions because of the difference in the

_____ during ventricular _____ and _____ .

Also, the P wave is _____ because _____ depolarization

doesn't occur.

    When electrical impulses are generated from the _____ instead of the

atria, _____ is lost and _____ decreases by as much as

_____ . Patients with ventricular arrhythmias may show signs and

symptoms of cardiac _____ , including _____ ,

_____ , _____ , and _____ distress.

    Although ventricular arrhythmias may be benign, they're potentially deadly because

the ventricles are ultimately responsible for _____ . Rapid recognition and

treatment of ventricular arrhythmias increase the chance for successful resuscitation.

Blanks numbered: 1, 2, 3, 4, 5, 6, 7, 8, 9, 10, 11, 12, 13, 14, 15, 16, 17, 18, 19, 20, 21, 22, 23, 24

Options

- 30%
- absent
- action potential
- angina
- atrial
- atrial kick
- bundle of His
- cardiac output
- decompensation
- depolarization
- depolarize
- hypotension
- myocardium
- opposite
- QRS complex
- repolarization
- respiratory
- syncope
- T wave
- ventricles

■ Strike out

Some of the statements below about ventricular arrhythmias are incorrect. Cross out the incorrect statements.

1. Premature ventricular contractions are usually caused by electrical irritability in the ventricular conduction system or muscle tissue.

2. Premature ventricular contractions rarely lead to more serious arrhythmias.

3. When a compensatory pause appears, the interval between two normal sinus beats containing a PVC equals two normal sinus intervals.

4. When a PVC strikes on the up slope of the preceding normal T wave, it's called the *R-on-T phenomenon*.

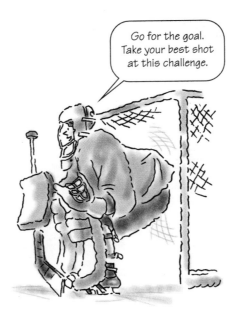

Go for the goal. Take your best shot at this challenge.

■ Fair or foul?

Can you identify the conditions that can disrupt electrolyte shifts and cause PVCs? Circle the conditions listed here that are correct.

1. Increased parasympathetic stimulation

2. Metabolic acidosis

3. Digoxin toxicity

4. Enlargement of the ventricular chambers

5. Caffeine or alcohol ingestion

You make the call

Interpret this rhythm strip by first describing the distinguishing characteristics and then identifying the arrhythmia.

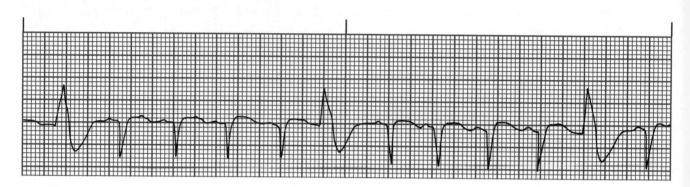

Rhythm: _____

Rate: _____

P wave: _____

PR interval: _____

QRS complex: _____

T wave: _____

QT interval: _____

Other: _____

Arrhythmia: _____

> It may be slow going at first, but keep trudging along and you'll see progress!

■ Cross-training

Complete this crossword puzzle using the clues below.

Across

2. A patient with PVCs will have a much _____ pulse wave after the premature beat

3. PVCs can stimulate retrograde P waves, which can _____ the ST segment

5. In patients with PVCs, the risk of developing a more serious arrhythmia increases with _____ hearts

8. As opposed to the timing of PVCs, this is when ventricular escape beats occur

10. Term for two PVCs in a row

12. On the ECG strip, PVCs appear as _____ beats

13. Term for three or more PVCs in a row

Down

1. A compensatory pause has a _____ baseline that follows the T wave of a PVC

4. Term used to describe PVCs that occur every third beat

6. Condition that can disrupt electrolyte shifts

7. A PVC is referred to as _____ when a compensatory pause doesn't occur

9. Premature beat occurring every other beat; alternates with normal QRS complexes

11. PVCs that look alike are considered this

Match point

PVCs can be very dangerous. See if you can match each pattern of PVCs listed below on the left with the correct strip on the right.

1. Paired PVCs _____

2. Multiform PVCs _____

3. Bigeminy _____

4. R-on-T phenomenon _____

A.
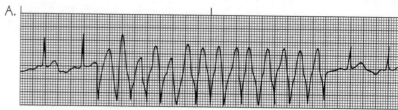

B.
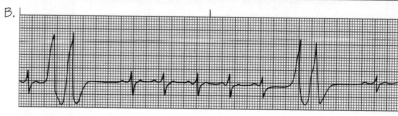

C.
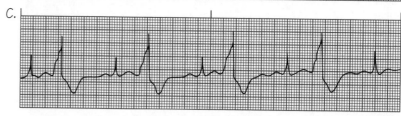

D.
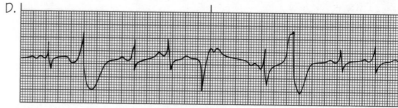

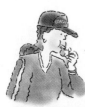

Coaching session
Deciphering PVCs

Is the rhythm you're assessing a premature ventricular contraction (PVC) or some other beat? How can you tell? You may be seeing ventricular escape beats or aberrantly conducted beats rather than PVCs. Escape beats act as a safety mechanism to protect the heart from ventricular standstill. The ventricular escape beat is late rather than premature. In addition, some supraventricular impulses take an abnormal pathway through the ventricular conduction system, causing the QRS complex to appear abnormal. These normal beats with aberrant ventricular conduction have P waves, whereas PVCs won't.

■■ Fair or foul?

Can you identify the characteristics of this idioventricular rhythm? Circle the characteristics that are correct.

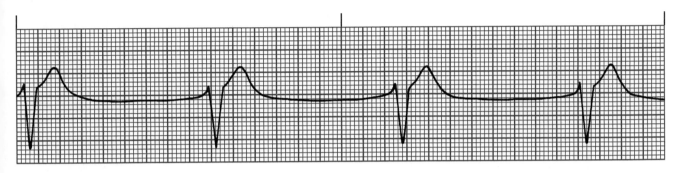

1. Rhythm: Regular

2. Rate: Unable to determine atrial rate; ventricular rate of 35 beats/minute

3. P wave: Follows QRS complex

4. PR interval: Unmeasurable

5. QRS complex: Wide and bizarre

6. T wave: Normal

7. QT interval: 0.30 second

8. Other: None

> Don't go off the deep end. Immerse yourself in this brain-boosting challenge.

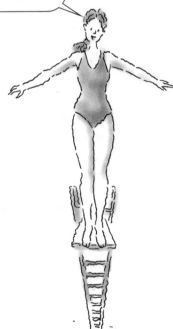

■■ Hit or miss

Some of the following statements about ventricular arrhythmias are true; the others are false. Label each one accordingly.

_____ 1. A patient with pulseless ventricular tachycardia receives the same treatment as one with ventricular fibrillation.

_____ 2. Any wide QRS complex tachycardia should be treated as idioventricular rhythm.

_____ 3. The cause of torsades de pointes is usually reversible.

_____ 4. In monomorphic ventricular tachycardia, the shape of the QRS complex constantly changes.

You make the call

Describe this device. When and why would it be used on a patient?

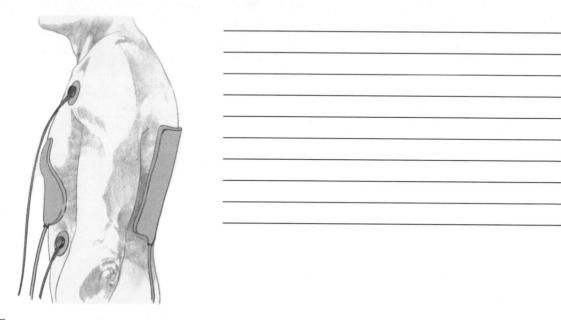

_____

_____

_____

_____

_____

_____

_____

_____

_____

_____

Jumble gym

Use the clues provided to help you unscramble terms related to ventricular arrhythmias. Then use the circled letters to answer the question below.

Question: Idioventricular rhythms should never be treated with which drug?

1. Compensatory pauses appear because the ventricle is in this phase

C A R T R Y E F O R   _ ◯ _ _ _ ◯ _ _ _ _

2. R-on-T phenomenon may interfere with this

T Z A R I N A L O O P I E R   _ _ _ _ ◯ _ _ _ _ _ _ _ _ _

3. A condition that can trigger PVCs

A D I O C Y L M R A   I M H A S I C E

_ _ ◯ _ _ _ ◯ _ _ _   ◯ _ _ _ _ _ _ _ ◯

4. Multiform PVCs indicate irritability here

L T E S E N V R C I   _ _ ◯ _ _ ◯ _ _ _ _

Answer: _ _ _ _ _ _ _ _ _ _

■ Match point

Match the treatment method on the left with the appropriate ventricular tachycardia on the right.

1. Administer amiodarone. Follow with synchronized cardioversion if necessary. _____

2. Administer magnesium. Load with 1 to 2 grams over 5 to 60 minutes. Follow with a magnesium infusion. _____

3. Deliver immediate synchronized cardioversion. _____

4. Seek expert consultation. _____

A. Recurrent polymorphic ventricular tachycardia

B. Stable ventricular tachycardia

C. Unstable ventricular tachycardia

D. Torsades de pointes

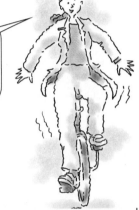

You show great talent. Continue practicing your technique on this rhythm strip.

■ You make the call

Interpret this rhythm strip by first describing the distinguishing characteristics and then identifying the arrhythmia.

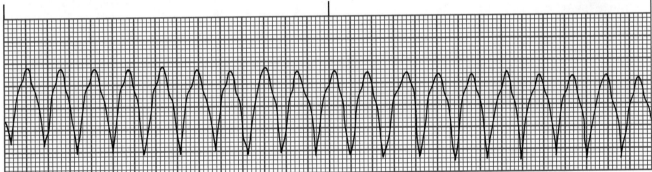

Rhythm: _____

Rate: _____

P wave: _____

PR interval: _____

QRS complex: _____

T wave: _____

QT interval: _____

Other: _____

Arrhythmia: _____

Cross-training

Still puzzled about ventricular arrhythmias? The clues in this crossword should help you figure them out.

Across

1. Another term for ventricular fibrillation
4. Can mimic ventricular fibrillation in patient
5. Drug that may help the heart respond better to defibrillation
7. With ventricular fibrillation, cardiac output falls to _____
10. Torsades de pointes is a special variation of this type of ventricular tachycardia
11. The rhythm of ventricular fibrillation

Down

2. In ventricular fibrillation, electrical impulses arise from many different _____
3. Until a defibrillator arrives, CPR should be performed to preserve the _____ supply to vital organs
4. The "S" in ACLS
6. Imbalance that can cause ventricular fibrillation
8. For treatment of ventricular fibrillation to be successful, response must be _____
9. The hallmark characteristic of torsades de pointes is QRS complexes that do this around the baseline

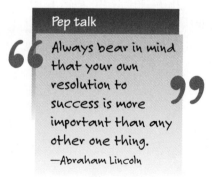

Pep talk

Always bear in mind that your own resolution to success is more important than any other one thing.
—Abraham Lincoln

■ Strike out

Some of the statements below are incorrect. Cross out the incorrect statements.

1. During defibrillation, the electrical current causes the myocardium to depolarize.

2. Ventricular fibrillation should never be treated with such drugs as amiodarone, lidocaine, procainamide, and magnesium sulfate.

3. Smaller (or fine) fibrillatory waves are easier to convert to a normal rhythm than are larger waves.

4. When treating ventricular fibrillation, vasopressin 40 units I.V. may be given to replace the first or second dose of epinephrine.

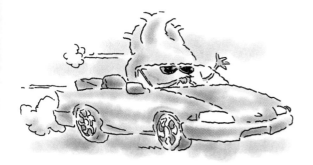

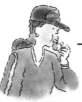

Coaching session

Torsades de pointes

Torsades de pointes is a special form of polymorphic ventricular tachycardia. QRS complexes that rotate about the baseline, deflecting downward and upward for several beats, are the distinguishing characteristic. The rate is 150 to 250 beats/minute, usually with an irregular rhythm. QRS complexes are wide with changing amplitude. The P wave is usually absent. When it occurs in children, torsades de pointes is usually due to congenital long QT syndrome.

■ Fair or foul?

Can you identify the characteristics of ventricular fibrillation? Circle the characteristics that are correct.

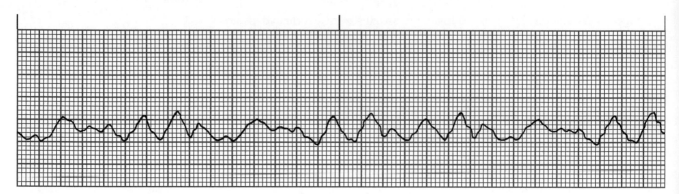

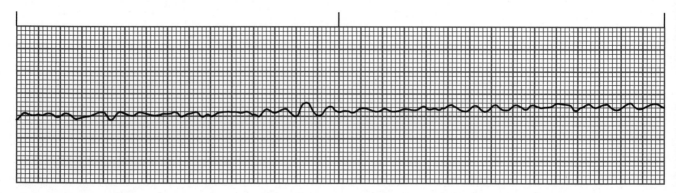

1. Rhythm: Irregular

2. Rate: Undetermined

3. P wave: Absent

4. PR interval: Unmeasurable

5. QRS complex: Wide and bizarre

6. T wave: Indiscernible

7. QT interval: Unmeasurable

8. Other: None

■■
■ Match point

Match each of the terms listed below on the left with the correct definition on the right.

1. Tension pneumothorax _____   A. Immediate treatment for asystole

2. Electric shock _____   B. Possible cause of pulseless electrical activity

3. Epinephrine _____   C. Drug used to treat pulseless electrical activity

4. Atropine _____   D. Possible cause of asystole

5. CPR _____   E. Drug used to treat patients with bradycardia

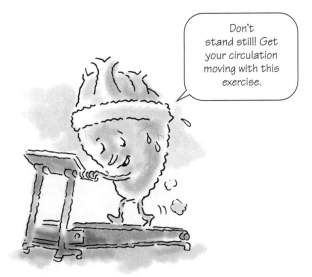

Don't stand still! Get your circulation moving with this exercise.

■■
■ Hit or miss

Some of the following statements are true; the others are false. Label each one accordingly.

_____ 1. In asystole, the patient will have no discernible pulse or blood pressure.

_____ 2. P waves may be present for a time on an ECG strip of a patient in asystole.

_____ 3. In pulseless electrical activity, there is no electrical activity in the heart and no cardiac output.

_____ 4. Pulseless electrical activity can lead to asystole.

Starting lineup

Put the following treatment steps in the order they should be performed on a patient with asystole.

Administer epinephrine, 1 mg I.V. push; repeat every 3 to 5 minutes.	1.
Assess airway, breathing, and circulation; then start CPR.	2.
Consider atropine, 1 mg I.V.; repeat every 3 to 5 minutes to a maximum of 0.04 mg/kg.	3.
Consider giving one dose of vasopressin 40 units I.V.	4.

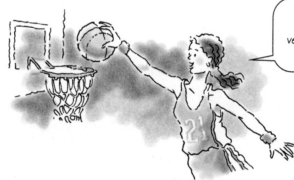

I hear you're a hot shot at analyzing ventricular arrhythmias. Analyze these!

Match point

Match each of these rhythm strips with the type of ventricular arrhythmia it shows.

1. _____

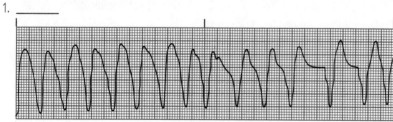

A. Ventricular fibrillation

B. Ventricular tachycardia

2. _____

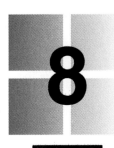

8

Atrioventricular blocks

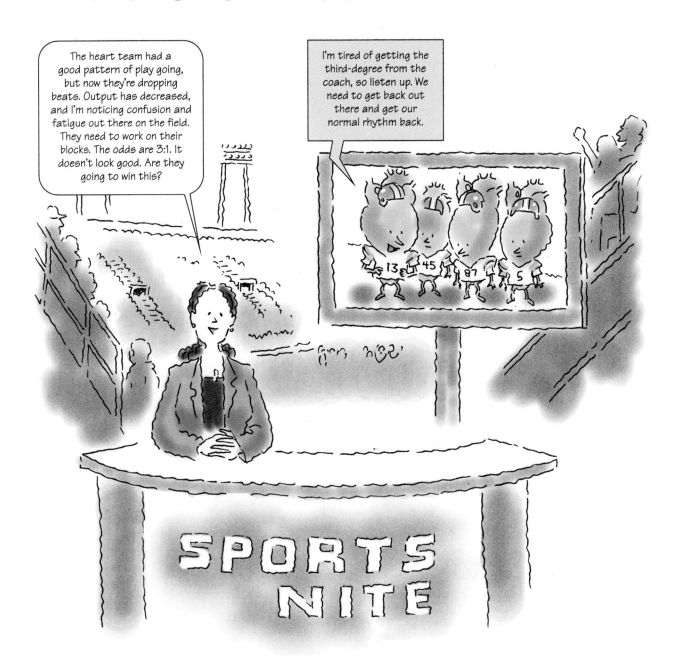

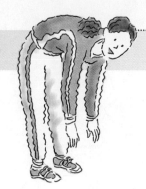

■■
■ Warm-up

Atrioventricular blocks review

AV blocks

■ Result from an interruption in impulse conduction between the atria and ventricles
■ Possibly occurring at the level of the atrioventricular (AV) node, the bundle of His, or the bundle branches
■ Atrial rate commonly normal (60 to 100 beats/minute) with slowed ventricular rate
■ Classified according to severity, not location

First-degree AV block

■ Occurs when impulses from the atria are consistently delayed during conduction through the AV node
■ Can progress to a more severe block

Characteristics

■ Electrocardiogram shows normal sinus rhythm except for prolonged PR interval
■ *Rhythm:* Regular
■ *P wave:* Normal
■ *PR interval:* Consistent for each beat; greater than 0.20 second
■ *QRS complex:* Normal; occasionally widened due to bundle-branch block
■ *QT interval:* Normal

Treatment

■ Correction of the underlying cause

Type I second-degree AV block

■ Also called *Mobitz type I block*

Characteristics

■ *Rhythm:* Atrial—regular; ventricular—irregular
■ *Rate:* Atrial rate exceeds ventricular rate
■ *P wave:* Normal
■ *PR interval:* Gradually gets longer with each beat until P wave fails to conduct to the ventricles
■ *QRS complex:* Usually normal
■ *T wave:* Normal

Treatment

■ No treatment if patient is asymptomatic
■ Atropine to improve AV conduction
■ Temporary pacemaker insertion

Type II second-degree AV block

■ Also known as *Mobitz type II block*
■ Occasional impulses from the sinoatrial (SA) node fail to conduct to the ventricles

Characteristics

■ *Rhythm:* Atrial—regular; ventricular—irregular if block is intermittent, regular if block is constant (such as 2:1 or 3:1)
■ *PR interval:* Constant for all conducted beats, may be prolonged in some cases
■ *QRS complex:* Usually wide
■ *T wave:* Normal
■ *Other:* PR and RR intervals constant before a dropped beat with no warning

Treatment

■ Temporary or permanent pacemaker insertion
■ Atropine, dopamine, or epinephrine for symptom-producing bradycardia
■ Discontinuation of digoxin if appropriate

Third-degree AV block

■ Also known as *complete heart block*
■ Impulses from the atria completely blocked at the AV node and not conducted to the ventricles

Characteristics

■ *Rhythm:* Atrial—regular; ventricular—regular
■ *Rate:* Atrial exceeds ventricular
■ *P wave:* Normal
■ *PR interval:* Varies with no regularity; no relation between P waves and QRS complexes
■ *QRS complex:* Normal (junctional pacemaker) or wide and bizarre (ventricular pacemaker)
■ *T wave:* Normal
■ *Other:* P waves without QRS complex

Treatment

■ Correction of the underlying cause
■ Temporary or permanent pacemaker
■ Atropine, dopamine, or epinephrine for symptom-producing bradycardia

Complete AV dissociation

- Atria and ventricles beat independently, each controlled by its own pacemaker

Characteristics

- *Rate:* Atrial and ventricular rates—nearly equal, with ventricular rate slightly faster
- *Rhythm:* Regular
- *PR interval:* No relation to QRS complex
- *QRS complex:* Usually normal; may be wide and bizarre

Treatment

- Correction of the underlying cause
- Atropine or isoproterenol to restore synchrony
- Pacemaker insertion

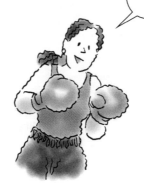

■ ■
■ Batter's box

Complete this fill-in-the-blank exercise to strengthen your knowledge of key concepts related to AV block.
Hint: Some words are used more than once.

AV block essentials

Atrioventricular heart block results from an _____ in the conduction of
                                                         1

impulses between the _____ and _____ . AV block can be
                               2   3

total or _____ or it may delay _____ . The block can
                 4   5

occur at the _____ , the _____ , or the
                    6   7

_____ .
        8

    The heart's electrical impulses normally originate in the _____ , so
                                                                              9

when those impulses are blocked at the _____ , atrial rates are
                                                  10

commonly normal (_____ to _____ beats/minute). The
                          11   12

clinical effect of the block depends on how many _____ are completely
                                                              13

blocked, how slow the _____ rate is as a result, and how the block
                              14

ultimately affects the _____ . A slow ventricular rate can decrease
                               15

cardiac output, possibly causing _____ , _____ , and
                                          16   17

_____ .
        18

    Various factors can lead to AV block, including underlying _____ ,
                                                                          19

use of certain _____ , congenital anomalies, and conditions that disrupt
                      20

the _____ system.
            21

Options
60
100
atria
AV node
bundle branches
bundle of His
cardiac conduction
conduction
confusion
drugs
heart
heart conditions
hypotension
impulses
interruption
light-headedness
partial
SA node
ventricles
ventricular

Sorry, can't stop now. I've got a rhythm going. I've got to stay consistent with the beat to keep my rate at target level.

■ Team up

Can you tell whether the causes below can create a temporary block or a permanent block? Place an "A" next to those that cause temporary block and a "B" next to those that cause permanent block. Be careful. Some may cause both types of blocks.

_____ 1. Digoxin toxicity

_____ 2. Cardiac surgery

_____ 3. Cardiomyopathy

_____ 4. Acute myocarditis

_____ 5. Calcium channel blockers

_____ 6. Beta-adrenergic blockers

_____ 7. Changes associated with aging

_____ 8. Anteroseptal myocardial infarction (MI)

_____ 9. Inferior wall MI

■ Cross-training

Complete this crossword puzzle using the clues below.

Across

1. First-degree AV block occurs when impulses from the atria are consistently _____ during conduction

4. Cause of first-degree AV block

7. A longer interval between S_1 and S_2 may be noted in a patient with first-degree block if the PR interval is this

8. If the conduction system isn't physically disrupted during cardiac surgery in which an AV block occurs, the block may only be _____

Down

2. Disruption of the conduction system can occur from a procedure called radiofrequency _____

3. AV blocks are classified according to this

5. Type of rhythm of first-degree AV block

6. If a portion of the conduction system is _____, a permanent block results

■ Match point

Match each of the rhythms on the left below with its characteristic on the right.

1. Third-degree AV block _____
2. Type I second-degree AV block _____
3. Type II second-degree AV block _____
4. First-degree AV block _____

A. PR interval gets progressively longer until a QRS complex is dropped
B. PR interval is constant but greater than 0.20 second
C. Atria and ventricles beat independently of each other
D. PR interval is constant for all conducted beats but QRS complexes are periodically missing

■ You make the call

Interpret this rhythm strip by first describing the distinguishing characteristics and then identifying the arrhythmia.

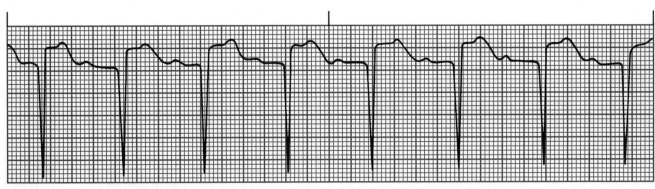

Rhythm: _____

Rate: _____

P wave: _____

PR interval: _____

QRS complex: _____

T wave: _____

QT interval: _____

Other: _____

Arrhythmia: _____

■ Hit or miss

Some of the following statements about type I second-degree AV block are true; the others are false. Label each one accordingly.

_____ 1. You should think of the phrase "longer, longer, drop" when identifying type I second-degree AV block.

_____ 2. The pattern of grouped beating seen in type I second-degree block is referred to as the footprints of Mobitz.

_____ 3. When caring for a symptomatic patient with type I second-degree block, no treatment is necessary.

_____ 4. The SA node isn't affected in a patient with type I second-degree AV block.

■ Jumble gym

Use the clues provided to help you unscramble terms related to type I second-degree AV block. Then use the circled letters to form a word that answers the question below.

Question: What's a possible symptom of type I second-degree block?

1. Most patients with type I second-degree AV block present with this finding

A P A T S Y C O M M I T _ ⃝⃝ _ ⃝ _ _ _ _ _ ⃝ _

2. Famous footprints sometimes used to describe type I second-degree AV block

A N W E B C H E C K _ ⃝⃝ _ _ _ _ _ _ ⃝

3. Drug that may be used to treat symptom-producing type I second-degree AV block

P I R A T E O N _ _ _ ⃝ _ _ ⃝ _

4. Famous name linked with second-degree block

B I Z T O M _ ⃝ _ _ ⃝ _

Answer: _ _ _ _ _ _ _ _ _ _ _

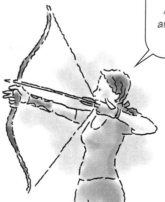

I know you aim to be the best at AV blocks. So here's another puzzle to help you hit the mark.

■ Fair or foul?

Can you identify the characteristics of type I second-degree AV block? Circle the characteristics that are correct.

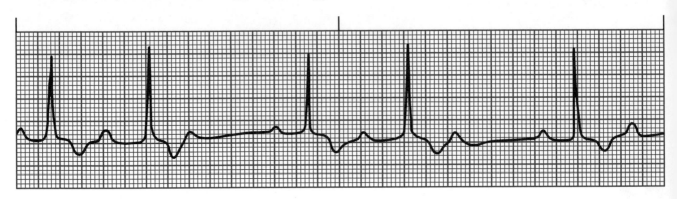

1. Rhythm: Atrial—regular; ventricular—irregular

2. Rate: Atrial—100 beats/minute; ventricular—60 beats/minute

3. P wave: Normal

4. PR interval: Unmeasurable

5. QRS complex: 0.08 second

6. T wave: Normal

7. QT interval: 0.36 second

8. Other: Wenckebach pattern of grouped beats

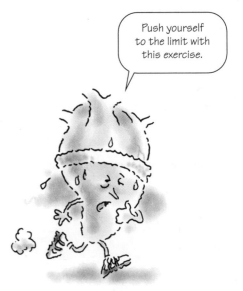

Push yourself to the limit with this exercise.

Match point

This exercise will test your knowledge of the patterns associated with common arrhythmias. Match each pattern with the corresponding rhythm type.

1. Grouped (as in type 1 second-degree AV block) _____

2. Normal, regular (as in normal sinus rhythm) _____

3. Premature (as in a premature ventricular contraction) _____

4. Paroxysm or burst (as in paroxysmal atrial tachycardia) _____

5. Slow, regular (as in sinus bradycardia) _____

6. Irregularly irregular (as in atrial fibrillation) _____

7. Fast, regular (as in sinus tachycardia) _____

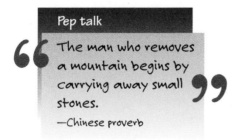

A.

B.

C.

D.

E.

F.

G.

Pep talk

" The man who removes a mountain begins by carrying away small stones. "

—Chinese proverb

■ You make the call

Using this sample rhythm strip as a guide, describe the distinguishing characteristics of high-grade AV block.

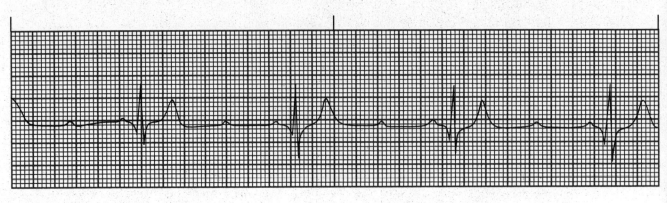

Rhythm: _____

Rate: _____

P wave: _____

PR interval: _____

QRS complex: _____

T wave: _____

QT interval: _____

Other: _____

■ Strike out

Some of the statements below about type II second-degree AV block are incorrect. Cross out the incorrect statements.

1. Type II block is more serious than type I because the ventricular rate tends to be slower and the cardiac output diminished.

2. In type II second-degree AV block, if the block is constant, such as 2:1 or 3:1, the rhythm is irregular.

3. When two or more successive ventricular impulses are blocked, the conduction disturbance is called high-grade atrioventricular block.

4. For patients with type II second-degree block who have signs of poor perfusion, transcutaneous pacing should be initiated.

■ Team up

Can you differentiate between type I second-degree AV block and type II second-degree AV block? Place an "A" next to the features common to type I second-degree AV block and a "B" next to those common to type II second-degree AV block.

_____ 1. The more common of the two blocks

_____ 2. The more serious of the two blocks

_____ 3. The PR interval gradually lengthens until a P wave eventually fails to appear

_____ 4. Has a constant PR interval but occasional P waves appear without a QRS complex

_____ 5. Reflects a problem at the bundle of His or bundle branches

_____ 6. Usually resolves with treatment of the underlying condition

■ Fair or foul?

Can you identify the characteristics of type II second-degree AV block? Circle the characteristics that are correct.

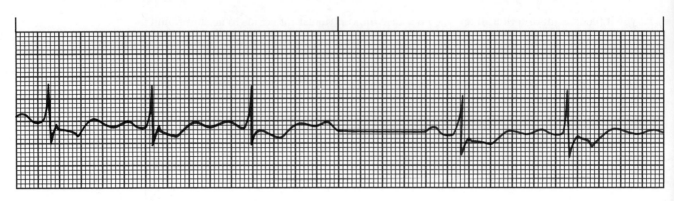

1. Rhythm: Atrial—regular; ventricular—irregular

2. Rate: Atrial—100 beats/minute; ventricular—60 beats/minute

3. P wave: Normal

4. PR interval: Unmeasurable

5. QRS complex: 0.10 second

6. T wave: Normal

7. QT interval: 0.45 second

8. Other: None

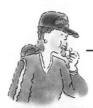

Coaching session
Heart block after congenital heart repair

A child may require a permanent pacemaker if complete heart block develops after repair of a ventricular septal defect. This arrhythmia may develop from interference with the bundle of His during surgery.

■ Cross-training

Assess your knowledge of AV block by completing this crossword puzzle.

Across

3. Third-degree AV block is also known as _____ heart block

4. If the patient's condition deteriorates, therapy aims to improve this rate

7. Third-degree AV block has a ventricular rhythm that typically originates from the _____ system

8. Until a permanent pacemaker can be inserted, temporary _____ may be required

Down

1. A symptom of third-degree heart block

2. Atrial kick is lost due to loss of _____ between the atrial and ventricular contractions

5. AV block that originates at the AV node level is most commonly caused by this kind of condition

6. Some relatively asymptomatic patients who have third-degree AV block complain that they can't tolerate this

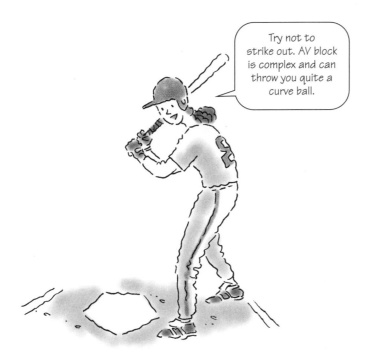

Try not to strike out. AV block is complex and can throw you quite a curve ball.

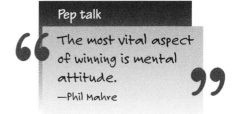

Pep talk

The most vital aspect of winning is mental attitude.

—Phil Mahre

■ You make the call

Interpret this rhythm strip by first describing the distinguishing characteristics and then identifying the arrhythmia.

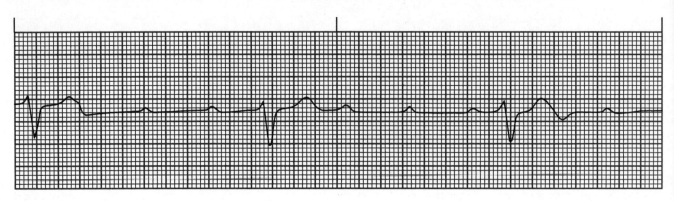

Rhythm: _____

Rate: _____

P wave: _____

PR interval: _____

QRS complex: _____

T wave: _____

QT interval: _____

Other: _____

Arrhythmia: _____

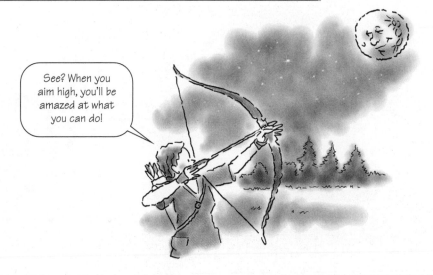

See? When you aim high, you'll be amazed at what you can do!

■ Team up

Can you determine which traits are common to third-degree AV block and which are common to complete AV dissociation? Place an "A" next to those that are common to third-degree block and a "B" next to those common to complete AV dissociation. Some traits may be common to both.

_____ 1. Can be caused by slowed sinus impulse formation or SA conduction, as in sinus bradycardia

_____ 2. The atrial and ventricular rates are about the same, with the ventricular rate slightly faster

_____ 3. Can be caused by calcium channel blockers

_____ 4. The atrial rate is faster than the ventricular rate

_____ 5. Can be caused by accelerated impulse formation in the AV junction, as in accelerated junctional tachycardia

_____ 6. Treatment may include isoproterenol

_____ 7. Can be caused by complete AV block

_____ 8. Treatment may include dopamine

_____ 9. The atria and ventricles beat independently, each controlled by its own pacemaker

_____ 10. Treatment may include placement of a pacemaker

■ Match point

A key as to which area of the heart is initiating an impulse may lie in its rate. Match the areas of the heart listed here with the rates they're capable of initiating.

1. SA node _____   A. 20 to 40 beats/minute

2. AV node _____   B. 60 to 100 beats/minute

3. Purkinje system _____   C. 40 to 60 beats/minute

■ Match point

Match each of these rhythm strips with the appropriate AV block in the right-hand column.

1. _____

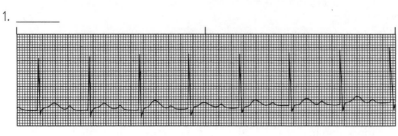

2. _____

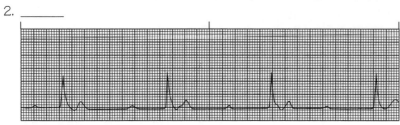

A. Third-degree AV block

B. Type II second-degree AV block

C. First-degree AV block

D. Complete AV dissociation

3. _____

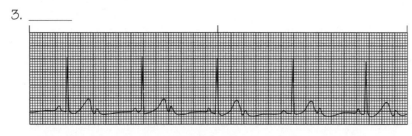

4. _____

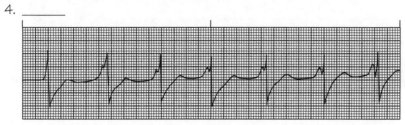

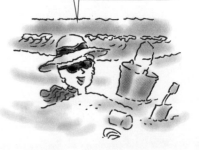

It's easy to get buried by all this information. Solve this last problem and you'll be able to take a well-deserved break.

9

Nonpharmacologic treatments

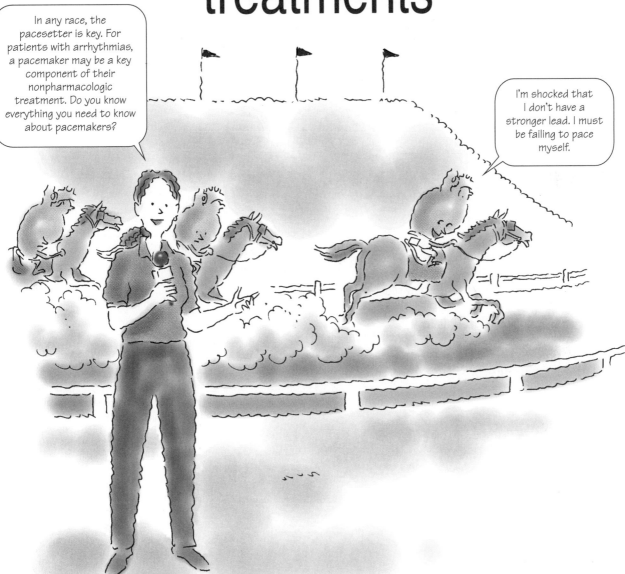

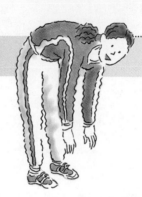

Nonpharmacologic treatment review

Pacemaker

- A device that electrically stimulates the myocardium to depolarize

Atrial and ventricular stimulation

- *Atria:* spike followed by a P wave and the patient's baseline QRS complex and T wave
- *Ventricles:* spike followed by a QRS complex and T wave
- *Atria and ventricles:* first spike followed by a P wave, then a spike, and then a QRS complex

Pacemaker codes

- First letter identifies the heart chambers being paced
- Second letter signifies the heart chamber sensed by the pacemaker
- Third letter refers to the pacemaker's response to the intrinsic electrical activity of the heart
- Fourth letter refers to the pacemaker's programmability
- Fifth letter refers to the pacemaker's response to a tachyarrhythmia

Pacemaker modes

- AAI: single-chambered pacemaker; paces and senses the atria
- VVI: paces and senses the ventricles
- DVI: paces both the atria and ventricles, only senses the ventricles
- DDD: fires when the ventricle doesn't respond on its own; paces the atria when the atrial rate falls below the lower set rate; senses and paces both atria and ventricles

Evaluating pacemakers

- Determine the pacemaker's mode and settings
- Review the patient's 12-lead electrocardiogram (ECG)
- Select a monitoring lead that clearly shows the pacemaker spikes
- Interpret the paced rhythm
- Look for information that tells which chamber is paced and about the pacemaker's sensing ability

Troubleshooting pacemakers

- Failure to capture: indicated by a spike without a complex
- Failure to pace: no pacemaker activity on the ECG
- Undersensing: help being given when none is needed
- Oversensing: won't pace when the patient actually needs it

Biventricular pacemaker

- Pacemaker has three leads: one to pace the right atrium, one to pace the right ventricle, and one to pace the left ventricle
- Both ventricles contract simultaneously, increasing cardiac output

Candidates

For treatment of patients with:
- class III and IV heart failure, with both systolic failure and ventricular dysynchrony
- symptom-producing heart failure despite maximal medical therapy
- QRS complex greater than 0.13 second
- left ventricular ejection fraction of 35% or less

Benefits of biventricular pacing

- Improves symptoms and activity tolerance
- Improves left ventricular remodeling and diastolic function and reduces sympathetic stimulation

Radiofrequency ablation

- Invasive procedure that uses radiofrequency energy to destroy heart tissue or conduction pathway responsible for arrhythmia
- Useful for atrial fibrillation and flutter, ventricular tachycardia (VT), atrioventricular (AV) nodal reentry tachycardia, and Wolff-Parkinson-White syndrome

Types of ablation

- Targeted ablation
- Pulmonary vein ablation
- AV nodal ablation (with pacemaker insertion)
- Accessory pathway ablation

Implantable cardioverter-defibrillator

- Also called an *ICD*
- Implanted device that monitors for bradycardia, VT, and ventricular fibrillation
- Provides shocks or paced beats to break arrhythmia

Types of therapy

- *Antitachycardia pacing:* bursts of pacing interrupt VT
- *Cardioversion:* shock timed to the R wave to terminate VT
- *Defibrillation:* shock to terminate ventricular fibrillation
- *Bradycardia pacing:* pacing when bradycardia is present

Programming information

- Type and model
- Status of the device (one or off)
- Therapies to be delivered (pacing, antitachycardia pacing, cardioversion, defibrillation)

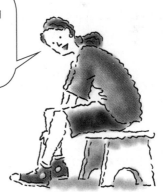

Now that you've limbered up your mental muscles, let's begin a workout designed to put you through your paces.

■ Boxing match

Fill in the answers to the clues below by using all of the syllables in the box. The number of syllables for each answer is shown in parentheses. Use each syllable only once. The first answer has been provided for you as an example.

~~AC~~	AL	ATRIO	~~CAR~~	CAR	CAR	CON	DE	~~DI~~
DI	DI	ED	ELEC	FARC	I	IM	IN	IZE
LAR	LAR	LITH	MYO	MYO	NUS	PLANT	PO	SI
SICK	TION	TION	TRAC	TRIC	TRODE	U	UM	UM
VEN								

1. Relating to the heart (3) C A R D I A C

2. Type of battery that provides power source for permanent pacemakers (3) _ _ _ _ _ _

3. A rhythmic, tightening action (3) _ _ _ _ _ _ _ _ _ _

4. Used to establish electrical contact (2) _ _ _ _ _ _ _ _

5. A sinoatrial (SA) node abnormality (3) _ _ _ _   _ _ _ _

6. The middle muscular layer of the heart wall (4) _ _ _ _ _ _ _ _ _

7. Heart attack (7) _ _ _ _ _ _ _ _ _ _
_ _ _ _ _ _ _ _

8. The myocardium's response to an electrical impulse (4) _ _ _ _ _ _ _ _ _

9. Situated between an atrium and a ventricle (5) _ _ _ _ _ _ _ _ _ _ _ _ _ _ _

10. Inserted permanently (3) _ _ _ _ _ _ _ _

■ Match point

Match each of the pacemaker spike descriptions below on the left to the appropriate pacemaker action on the right.

1. The spike is followed by a QRS complex and a T wave. The QRS complex appears wider than the patient's own QRS complex. _____

2. The spike is followed by a P wave and the patient's baseline QRS complex and T wave. The P wave may look different from the patient's normal P wave.

_____

3. The first spike is followed by a P wave, then a spike, and then a QRS complex. _____

A. Atria are stimulated by the pacemaker.

B. Ventricles are stimulated by the pacemaker.

C. Both atria and ventricles are stimulated by the pacemaker.

■ Cross-training

Complete this crossword puzzle using the clues below to test your knowledge of pacemakers.

Across

1. Interior muscle ridge
6. Type of pacemaker used to treat chronic AV block
9. Type of temporary pacemaker used for patients undergoing cardiac surgery
11. Measurement of pacemaker's sensing threshold
12. Type of lead system that's more sensitive to the heart's intrinsic activity
13. Microchip in a pulse generator that guides heart pacing

Down

2. The stimulation threshold is sometimes referred to as the energy required for

   _____

3. Type of pacemaker commonly used in an emergency
4. Number of years the battery in a permanent pacemaker usually lasts
5. Area under which permanent pacemaker pocket is constructed
7. The most common and reliable type of temporary pacemaker
8. Where permanent pacemaker leads are anchored
10. Type of pacing lead that contains the positive pole within the lead

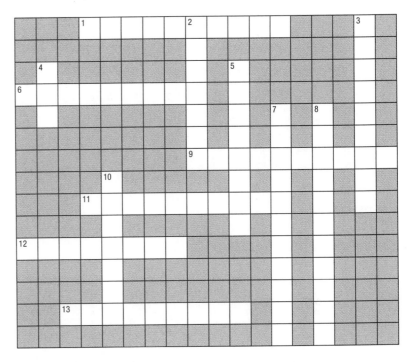

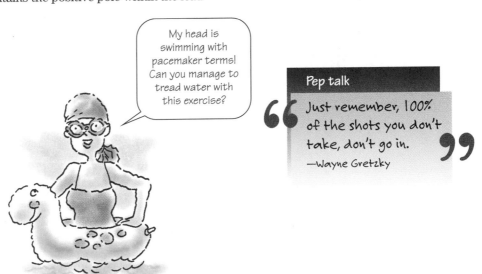

My head is swimming with pacemaker terms! Can you manage to tread water with this exercise?

Pep talk

Just remember, 100% of the shots you don't take, don't go in.
—Wayne Gretzky

■ Strike out

Some of the statements below about pacemakers are incorrect. Cross out the incorrect statements.

1. Pacemaker spikes appear above or below the isoelectric line.

2. On an ECG, a pacemaker spike occurs when the pacemaker sends an electrical impulse to the SA node.

3. Lead placement for a pacemaker is dependent on the age of the patient.

4. A permanent pacemaker is usually programmed before implantation.

■ Match point

Match each pacemaker mode on the left below with its corresponding rhythm on the right.

1. AAI _____

2. VVI _____

3. DVI _____

4. DDD _____

> Ready to jump into pacemaker codes? It will take some high steppin' to decipher these.

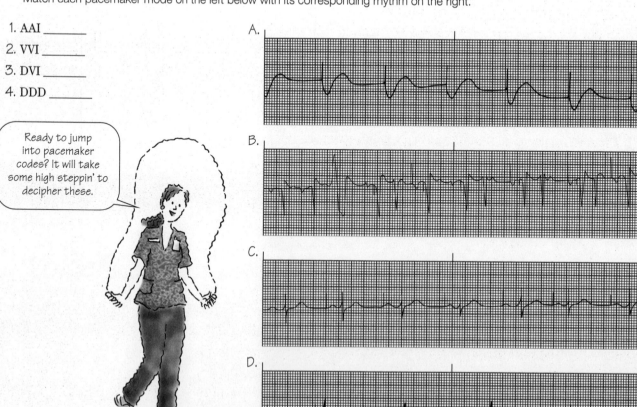

■ Hit or miss

Some of the following statements about pacemakers are true; the others are false. Label each one accordingly.

_____ 1. One of the benefits of DDD mode is the ability to change modes automatically.

_____ 2. AAI pacemaker mode is commonly used in AV block.

_____ 3. DVI pacemaker mode won't adjust its rate for active patients.

_____ 4. A committed DVI pacemaker generates an impulse even with spontaneous ventricular depolarization.

_____ 5. DDD mode benefits patients by maintaining AV synchrony.

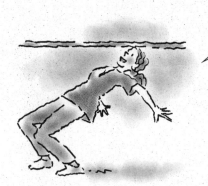

Flex your mind and your muscles with this workout.

■ Starting lineup

Put the following steps for determining whether your patient's pacemaker is functioning properly in the correct order.

Review the patient's 12-lead ECG.
Interpret the ECG tracing's paced rhythm and compare with patient's pacemaker.
Look for information that tells you which chamber is paced and the pacemaker's sensing ability.
Determine the pacemaker's mode and settings.
Select a monitoring lead that shows the pacemaker spikes.

1.

2.

3.

4.

5.

■ Team up

See if you can determine which corrective actions should be taken with each pacemaker malfunction. Mark each action appropriately: Write an "A" for "Failure to capture," a "B" for "Failure to pace," and a "C" for "Failure to sense intrinsic beats." Be careful! Some may have more than one answer.

_____ 1. Remove items in the room that might cause electromechanical interference.

_____ 2. Change the battery or pulse generator.

_____ 3. Turn the sensitivity control to a lower number.

_____ 4. Increase the milliampere setting slowly.

_____ 5. Check the connections to the cable and the position of the pacing electrode in the patient.

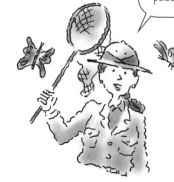

Don't let your mind flit about. Focus on these pacemaker terms.

■ You make the call

Can you correctly identify the pacemaker malfunctions reflected by the sample rhythm strips shown below? For each strip, identify the malfunction and how that malfunction is revealed on an ECG.

1.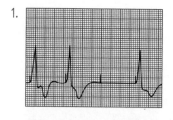

_____
_____
_____
_____
_____

2.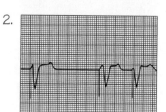

_____
_____
_____
_____
_____

3.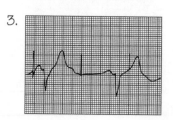

_____
_____
_____
_____
_____

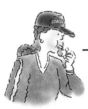

Coaching session
When a pacemaker malfunctions

How you intervene when a pacemaker malfunctions depends on the nature of the problem. Follow these guidelines.

Failure to capture
• If the patient's condition has changed, notify the doctor.
• Be sure the pacemaker settings are correct.
• Check all of the connections.

Failure to pace
• If the pacing or indicator light is flashing, check the connections.
• If the pulse generator is turned on but the indicators aren't flashing, change the battery. If that doesn't help, change the generator.

Failure to sense intrinsic beats
• If the pacemaker is undersensing, turn the sensitivity control completely to the right (to a smaller number). If the pacemaker is oversensing, turn the control slightly to the left.
• Change the battery or pulse generator.
• Remove any items in the room that may cause electromechanical interference.
• If the pacemaker still fires on the T wave, turn it off (per facility policy). Make sure atropine is available and be prepared to initiate cardiopulmonary resuscitation.

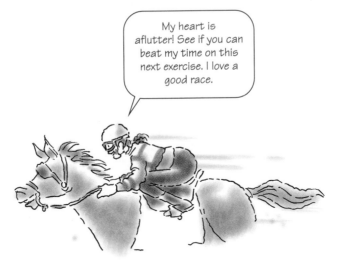

My heart is aflutter! See if you can beat my time on this next exercise. I love a good race.

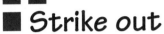
Strike out

Some of the statements below about biventricular pacemakers are incorrect. Cross out the incorrect statements.

1. Biventricular pacemakers have two leads: one to pace the right atrium and one to pace the right ventricle.

2. Biventricular pacing improves left ventricular remodeling and diastolic function and reduces sympathetic stimulation.

3. Biventricular pacing may be used in the treatment of patients with class III and IV heart failure.

4. The electrode tip for the right ventricle is placed in the coronary sinus to a branch of the inferior cardiac vein.

5. In order to benefit from biventricular pacing, candidates should have both systolic heart failure and ventricular dysynchrony.

Cross-training

Radiofrequency ablation is an invasive procedure that may be used when a patient with an arrhythmia hasn't responded to antiarrhythmic drugs or cardioversion. Complete this crossword puzzle to test your knowledge of radiofrequency ablation.

Across

6. When caring for a patient after radiofrequency ablation, check the catheter insertion site for _____ formation

8. Means used to deliver the radiofrequency energy to the heart tissue

9. Anticoagulation therapy may be needed to reduce this risk

10. Radiofrequency ablation is used to destroy the focus of an arrhythmia or _____ the conduction pathway

11. The radiofrequency ablation procedure can be _____

12. When this is the cause of the arrhythmia, ablation can destroy the pathway without affecting the AV node

Down

1. Atrial _____ is one condition that radiofrequency ablation is effective in treating

2. Following ablation of the AV node, the patient may need one of these

3. In some patients, the tissue inside the _____ vein is responsible for the arrhythmia

4. Besides radiofrequency, another type of energy that can be used to destroy heart tissue

5. Vein commonly used to insert ablation catheter

7. Electrophysiology studies _____ the area causing the arrhythmia

Pep talk

"Anytime you suffer a setback or disappointment, put your head down and plow ahead."
—Les Brown

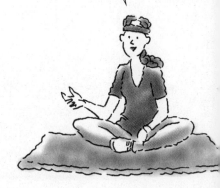

A trained mind can concentrate when it needs to.

■ Jumble gym

Unscramble the following words to discover the names of arrhythmias effectively treated by radiofrequency ablation. Then use the circled letters to form a word that answers the question below.

Question: If atrial fibrillation isn't terminated by targeted ablation, what type of AV ablation may be used to block electrical impulses from being conducted to the ventricles?

1. ALTARI LETTURF _ _ _ _ _ _ _ O _ _ _ _ _

2. CURRANTVILE CICADAHATRY _ _ O _ _ _ _ _ _ _ _ _
_ _ _ _ _ _ _ _ _ _

3. VA LADON TERNRYE _ _ _ _ O _ _ _ _ _ _ _ _ _

4. YACHTCARADI _ O _ _ _ _ _ _ _ _ _

5. FLOW-APRONSINK-HEWIT DRYOMENS
_ _ _ _ - _ _ _ _ _ _ _ _ _ _ - _ _ _ _ _ _ _ _ _ _ _ O _ _

Answer: _ _ _ _ _ _

■ Hit or miss

Some of the following statements about ICD therapy are true; the others are false. Label each one accordingly.

_____ 1. A patient with an ICD who's experiencing cardiac arrest should be treated with dopamine.

_____ 2. An ICD consists of a programmable pulse generator and one or more lead wires.

_____ 3. Watch for signs of a perforated ventricle, with resultant cardiac tamponade. Signs include fatigue and blurred vision.

_____ 4. An ICD provides continuous monitoring of the heart for bradycardia, VT, and ventricular fibrillation.

■ Match point

Match the type of ICD therapy on the left with its definition on the right.

1. Antitachycardia pacing _____

2. Cardioversion _____

3. Defibrillation _____

4. Bradycardia pacing _____

A. A low- or high- energy shock is timed to the R wave to terminate VT and return the heart to its normal rhythm.

B. A high-energy shock to the heart is used to terminate ventricular fibrillation and return the heart to its normal rhythm.

C. A series of small, rapid, electrical pacing pulses are used to interrupt VT and return the heart to its normal rhythm.

D. Electrical pacing pulses are used when the heart's natural electrical signals are too slow.

■ Finish line

Using the illustration below, identify the parts—and the function of each part—of a single-chamber temporary pulse generator.

1. _____
   _____

2. _____
   _____

3. _____
   _____

4. _____
   _____
   _____

5. _____
   _____

6. _____

7. _____
   _____
   _____

8. _____
   _____

9. _____
   _____

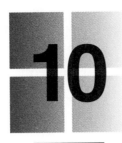

Pharmacologic treatment

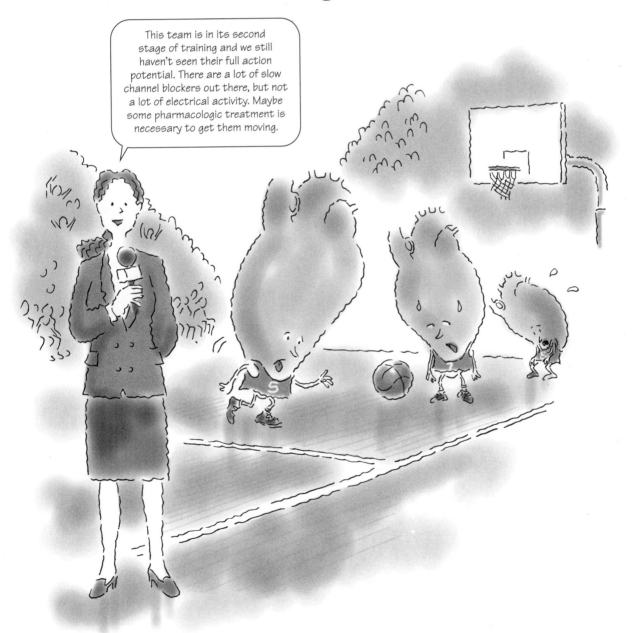

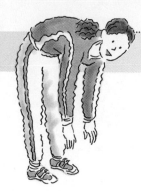

Pharmacologic treatment review

Antiarrhythmic drugs

▪ Classified according to effect on the cell's electrical activity (action potential) and mechanism of action

Class Ia antiarrhythmics

▪ Also called *sodium channel blockers*
▪ Reduce excitability of cardiac cells and decrease contractility
▪ Have anticholinergic and proarrhythmic effects
▪ Show widened QRS complex and prolonged QT intervals on electrocardiogram (ECG)

QUINIDINE

▪ Used for supraventricular and ventricular arrhythmias

PROCAINAMIDE HYDROCHLORIDE

▪ Used for supraventricular and ventricular arrhythmias

Class Ib antiarrhythmics

▪ Suppress ventricular ectopy
▪ Slow phase 0 depolarization
▪ Shorten phase 3 repolarization and action potential

LIDOCAINE HYDROCHLORIDE

▪ Former drug of choice for suppressing ventricular arrhythmias

TOCAINAMIDE HYDROCHLORIDE

▪ Suppresses life-threatening ventricular arrhythmias

Class Ic antiarrhythmics

▪ Slow conduction

FLECAINIDE ACETATE

▪ Used for paroxysmal atrial fibrillation or flutter in patients without structural heart disease and with life-threatening ventricular arrhythmias; prevents supraventricular tachycardia

PROPAFENONE HYDROCHLORIDE

▪ Used only for life-threatening ventricular arrhythmias

Class II antiarrhythmics

▪ Also called *beta-adrenergic blockers*
▪ Block sympathetic nervous system beta receptors and decrease heart rate
▪ Used to treat supraventricular and ventricular arrhythmias
▪ Include acebutolol, propranolol, esmolol, and sotalol

Class III antiarrhythmics

▪ Also called *potassium channel blockers*
▪ Block potassium movement during phase 3
▪ Increase the duration of the action potential
▪ Prolong the effective refractory period
▪ Show prolonged PR and QT intervals and widened QRS complex on ECG

AMIODARONE

▪ Used for supraventricular arrhythmias, paroxysmal supraventricular tachycardia (PSVT) caused by accessory pathway conduction (as in Wolff-Parkinson-White syndrome), and ventricular arrhythmias

IBUTILIDE FUMARATE

▪ Rapidly converts recent-onset atrial fibrillation or flutter

DOFETILIDE

▪ Maintains normal sinus rhythm in patients with atrial fibrillation or flutter lasting longer than 1 week, who have been converted to normal sinus rhythm
▪ Used to convert atrial fibrillation and flutter to normal sinus rhythm

Class IV antiarrhythmics

▪ Also called *calcium channel blockers*
▪ Prolong conduction time and refractory period in the atrioventricular (AV) node
▪ Decrease contractility
▪ Show PR interval prolonged on ECG

VERAPAMIL

▪ Used for PSVT and to slow ventricular response in atrial fibrillation and flutter

DILTIAZEM

▪ Used for PSVT and atrial fibrillation or flutter

Unclassified antiarrhythmics

ADENOSINE
- Slows AV node conduction and inhibits reentry pathways
- Used to treat PSVT

ATROPINE
- Anticholinergic drug that blocks vagal effects on the sino-atrial (SA) and AV nodes
- Used to treat symptomatic bradycardia and asystole

DIGOXIN
- Enhances vagal tone and slows conduction through the SA and AV nodes
- Shows ST-segment depression opposite the QRS deflection on ECG; P wave may be notched
- Used to treat PSVT and atrial fibrillation and flutter

EPINEPHRINE
- Catecholamine that acts on alpha-adrenergic and beta-adrenergic receptor sites of the sympathetic nervous system
- Used for symptomatic bradycardia and to restore cardiac rhythm in cardiac arrest

MAGNESIUM SULFATE
- Decreases cardiac cell excitability and conduction; slows conduction through the AV node and prolongs the refractory period
- Used to treat ventricular arrhythmias

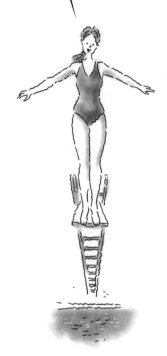

A good workout is just the thing to keep your mental muscles strong. Ready? Let's dive in!

■ Match point

Match each of the antiarrhythmic classes below on the left with its effect on the heart's action potential.

1. Class Ia _____
2. Class Ib _____
3. Class Ic _____
4. Class IV _____

A. Markedly slows phase 0 depolarization and reduces conduction (used only for refractory arrhythmias)

B. Prolongs conductivity and increases the refractory period at the AV node; also called slow channel blockers

C. Reduces conductivity and prolongs repolarization and the action potential

D. Slows phase 0 depolarization, doesn't affect conductivity, and shortens phase 3 repolarization and the action potential

■ Hit or miss

Some of the following statements about antiarrhythmic drugs are true; the others are false. Label each one accordingly.

_____ 1. Class Ia antiarrhythmic drugs include quinidine and procainamide.

_____ 2. Quinidine is used to treat patients with supraventricular and ventricular arrhythmias.

_____ 3. Adverse cardiovascular effects of quinidine include pericarditis, thrombosis, and bradycardia.

_____ 4. Quinidine should be avoided in patients with first-degree AV block.

_____ 5. You should notify the doctor if the QRS complex of a patient on quinidine therapy widens by 25% or more.

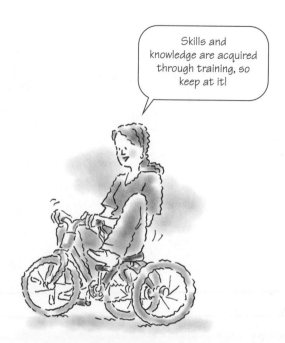

Skills and knowledge are acquired through training, so keep at it!

■ Jumble gym

Unscramble the words to uncover adverse effects related to the antiarrhythmic drug procainamide. Then use the circled letters to answer the question.

Question: Patients taking procainamide should have their serum drug levels monitored as well as their level of which active metabolite? (*Hint:* The answer is an abbreviation.)

1. E A U N A S ◯ _ _ _ _ _

2. A C R I B A Y D R A D _ _ ◯ _ _ _ _ _ _ _ _

3. L S E Y A O S T ◯ _ _ _ _ _ _ _

4. H O N E Y P I S T O N _ _ ◯ _ _ _ _ _ _ _

Answer: _ _ _ _

■ Strike out

Some of the statements below about antiarrhythmic drugs are incorrect. Cross out the incorrect statements.

1. Class 1b antiarrhythmics are effective in suppressing supraventricular arrhythmias.

2. One factor that may increase a patient's potential for lidocaine toxicity is taking the drug cimetidine or propranolol.

3. Lidocaine is the drug of choice in suppressing ventricular arrhythmias.

4. Cardiovascular adverse effects of lidocaine include AV block, hypotension, bradycardia, new or worsened arrhythmias, and cardiac arrest.

5. Lidocaine should be avoided in patients with severe SA, AV, or intraventricular block who do not have artificial pacemakers.

Memory jogger

To remember what each of the four classifications if anti-arrhythmic drugs blocks, think "Sure Beats Picking Corn":

- Class I: S_____
- Class II: B_____
- Class III: P_____
- Class IV: C_____

■ Cross-training

Complete this crossword puzzle using the clues below.

Across

2. Trade name of propafenone

4. Organ responsible for changing most drugs into active or inactive metabolites

5. In a patient taking flecainide, report _____ of the QRS complex by 25% or more

7. Propafenone should be used cautiously with this anticoagulant

11. Adverse effect of flecainide to the central nervous system

12. Trade name of flecainide

Down

1. Class 1c antiarrhythmics slow _____ without effecting the duration of the action potential

3. The calcium channel is also called the _____ channel

6. This imbalance should be corrected before starting flecainide

8. Hematologic adverse effect of propafenone

9. Class 1c antiarrhythmics block the influx of this during phase 0

10. The sodium channel is also called the _____ channel

Pep talk

"Unless you try to do something beyond what you have already mastered, you will never grow."

—Ronald Osborn

■ Match point

Match each of the following beta-adrenergic blockers below with its correct classification and characteristics.

1. Acebutolol _____
2. Propranolol _____
3. Esmolol _____
4. Sotalol _____

A. Noncardioselective; decreases heart rate, contractility, and blood pressure; and reduces the incidence of sudden cardiac death after MI

B. Short-acting, cardioselective drug that decreases heart rate, contractility, and blood pressure; administered by I.V. titration

C. Cardioselective and decreases contractility, heart rate, and blood pressure

D. Noncardioselective; decreases heart rate, slows AV conduction, decreases cardiac output, and lowers systolic and diastolic blood pressure

■ Hit or miss

Some of the following statements about beta-adrenergic blockers are true; the others are false. Label each one accordingly.

_____ 1. Beta$_2$ receptors relax smooth muscle in the bronchi and blood vessels.

_____ 2. Beta-adrenergic blockers that block both beta$_1$ and beta$_2$ are referred to as *noncardioselective*.

_____ 3. Beta$_1$ receptors decrease heart rate, contractility and conductivity.

_____ 4. Beta-adrenergic blockers block beta receptors in the parasympathetic nervous system.

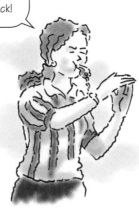

■ Mind sprints

Go the distance by listing as many adverse effects of beta-adrenergic blockers as you can in 3 minutes. Remember that beta-adrenergic blockers can have not only adverse cardiovascular effects but also central nervous system, respiratory, hematologic, and integumentary effects.

1. _____
2. _____
3. _____
4. _____
5. _____
6. _____
7. _____
8. _____
9. _____
10. _____

11. _____
12. _____
13. _____
14. _____
15. _____
16. _____
17. _____
18. _____
19. _____
20. _____

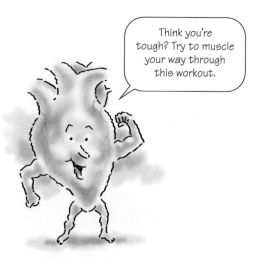

Think you're tough? Try to muscle your way through this workout.

■ Team up

Can you determine to which class of antiarrhythmics the following effects belong? Label each of the effects below as class Ia, Ib, Ic, or II. Be careful because some may have more than one answer.

_____ 1. Suppresses ventricular automaticity in ischemic tissue

_____ 2. Depresses sinoatrial node automaticity

_____ 3. Prolongs repolarization and the duration of the action potential

_____ 4. Shortens the duration of the action potential

_____ 5. Decreases contractility

_____ 6. Inhibits sympathetic activity

Power stretch

The effects of antiarrhythmic drugs on the cardiac cycle lead to specific ECG changes. First, in the left column, match each antiarrhythmic drug class with its specific ECG effects, listed below. (*Hint:* The effects listed may apply to more than one class.) Next, in the right column, stretch your knowledge further by labeling each ECG strip with the drug class responsible for the ECG changes shown in that strip.

1. Class 1a _____

2. Class 1b _____

3. Class 1c _____

4. Class II _____

A. Prolongs the PR interval

B. Prolongs the QT interval

C. Shortens the QT interval

D. Widens the QRS complex

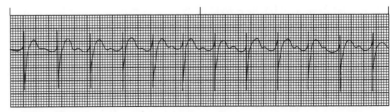

Rhythm strip 1 _____

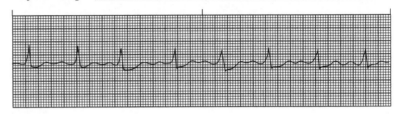

Rhythm strip 2 _____

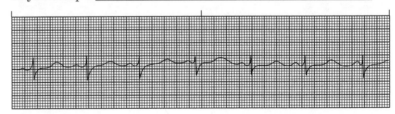

Rhythm strip 3 _____

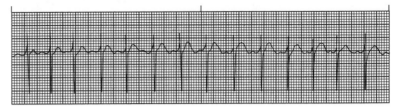

Rhythm strip 4 _____

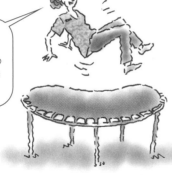

You rebounded well after that last challenge. Can you do the same with these ECG strips?

■ Strike out

Some of the statements below about class III antiarrhythmics are incorrect. Cross out the incorrect statements.

1. Long-term dofetilide therapy is associated with vision disturbances.

2. All class III antiarrhythmics have proarrhythmic potential.

3. Amiodarone can be used to treat Wolff-Parkinson-White syndrome.

4. Ibutilide fumarate shouldn't be administered at the same time or within 4 hours of class 1b antiarrhythmics.

5. Patients undergoing amiodarone treatment should wear sunscreen and protective clothing to avoid photosensitivity reactions.

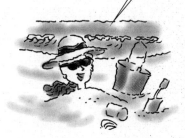

It's nice to bask in the sun after a long workout, but if you're taking amiodarone, you shouldn't disregard SA block, AV block, and sunblock!

■ Mind sprints

Go the distance by listing as many nursing considerations for amiodarone administration as you can in 3 minutes.

1. _____

2. _____

3. _____

4. _____

5. _____

6. _____

7. _____

8. _____

9. _____

10. _____

Jumble gym

Use the clues provided to help you unscramble terms related to class IV antiarrhythmics. Then use the circled letters to answer the question below.

Question: You should be cautious when administering diltiazem to which patients?

1. Prolong this phase of the cardiac cycle

E Y R T O F A R C R   D O P R I E

_ _ _ _ _ _ _ _ _〇 _ _ _ _ _〇

2. Condition commonly treated by drugs in this group

O Y S E N H E N T P R I   _ _ _〇_ _〇_ _ _ _ _

3. Drug used to treat PSVT

R M I A V L E P A   _ _〇_ _ _〇_ _

4. Specific channel blocked by these drugs

U M C C L A I   _ _〇_ _ _ _

Answer: _ _ _ _ _ _ _

> Don't pitch your hopes too high. It will take time and effort to build mastery of arrhythmias.

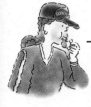

Coaching session
Drug metabolism and elimination across the life span

Neonates have a reduced ability to metabolize drugs because of the limited activity of liver enzymes at the time of birth. As infants grow, drug metabolism improves. Glomerular filtration rate is also reduced at birth, causing neonates to eliminate drugs more slowly than adults.

In older patients, advancing age usually reduces the blood supply to the liver and certain liver enzymes become less active. Consequently, the liver loses some of its ability to metabolize drugs. With reduced liver function, higher drug levels remain in circulation, causing more intense drug effects and increasing the risk of drug toxicity. Because kidney function also diminishes with age, drug elimination may be impaired, resulting in increased drug levels.

■ Hit or miss

Some of the following statements about unclassified antiarrhythmic drugs are true; the others are false.
Label each one accordingly.

_____ 1. Adenosine is used to treat symptom-producing bradycardia and asystole.

_____ 2. Atropine is ineffective in patients following dissection of the vagus nerve during heart transplant surgery.

_____ 3. Digoxin weakens myocardial contraction.

_____ 4. Epinephrine increases systolic blood pressure.

_____ 5. Magnesium sulfate shouldn't be administered to patients with renal insufficiency.

■ Team up

Can you determine to which class of antiarrhythmics the following effects belong? Label each of the effects as class III or
class IV, as appropriate.

_____ 1. Blocks calcium movement during phase 2

_____ 2. Increases duration of the action potential

_____ 3. Decreases contractility

_____ 4. Blocks potassium movement during phase 3

_____ 5. Prolongs the effective refractory period

_____ 6. Prolongs the conduction time and increases the refractory period in the AV node

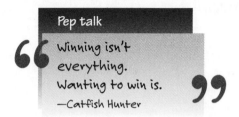

Pep talk

“ Winning isn't
everything.
Wanting to win is.
—Catfish Hunter ”

Cross-training

Some antiarrhythmic drugs defy classification. Use the clues below to complete this crossword puzzle about unclassified antiarrhythmic drugs.

Across

4. Epinephrine shouldn't be mixed with these solutions
5. Adverse cardiovascular effect of magnesium sulfate
7. Drug that enhances vagal tone and slows conduction through the SA and AV nodes
8. Effect caused by too much digoxin in the body
9. Adverse effect of adenosine; short _____ pause at the time of conversion

Down

1. Condition for which atropine shouldn't be used unless the patient is symptomatic
2. Drug that acts directly on alpha- and beta- adrenergic receptor sites of the sympathetic nervous system
3. Types of effects atropine blocks on the SA and AV nodes
4. Naturally occurring nucleoside
6. Magnesium sulfate decreases myocardial cell excitability and _____

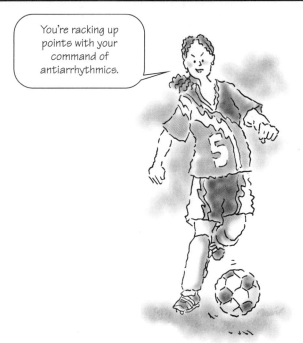

You're racking up points with your command of antiarrhythmics.

Power stretch

The effects of antiarrhythmic drugs on the cardiac cycle lead to specific ECG changes. First, in the left column, match each antiarrhythmic drug class with its specific ECG effects, listed below. Next, in the right column, stretch your knowledge further by labeling each ECG strip with the drug class responsible for the ECG changes shown in that strip.

1. Class III _____

2. Class IV _____

3. Digoxin _____

A. Enhances vagal tone (slowing heart rate)

B. Shortens the action potential, which shortens refractoriness

C. Blocks potassium movement during phase 3 of action potential

D. Blocks calcium movement during phase 2 of action potential

E. Produces gradual sloping of ST segment, causing ST-segment depression in the direction opposite that of the QRS

F. Prolongs conduction time (leading to a decreased atrial and ventricular rate)

G. May cause notched P wave

H. Increases the refractory period in the AV node (causing a prolonged PR interval)

I. Increases the duration of the action potential

J. Prolongs the refractory period (leading to a prolonged PR interval and a prolonged QT interval)

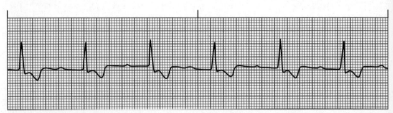

Rhythm strip 1 _____

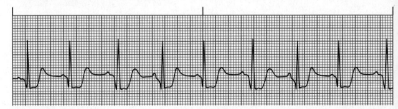

Rhythm strip 2 _____

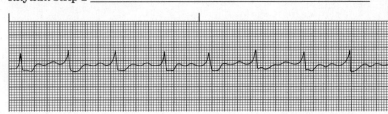

Rhythm strip 3 _____

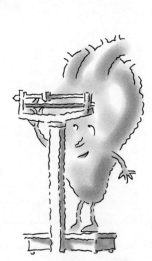

Patients taking antiarrhythmics should report any unusual weight changes to their doctors.

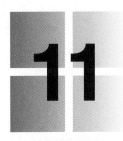

Obtaining a 12-lead ECG

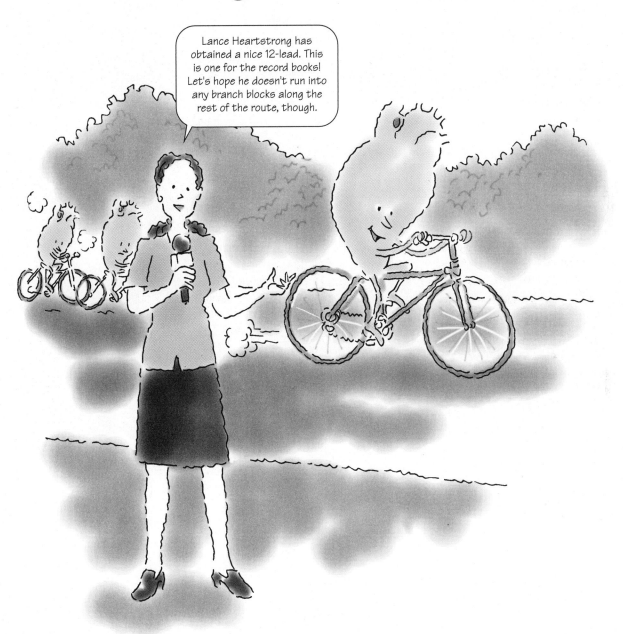

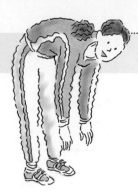

▪▪ **Warm-up**

Obtaining a 12-lead ECG review

12-lead ECG basics

▪ Provides 12 different views of the heart's electrical activity

The limb leads

▪ Three bipolar limb leads: I, II, and III
▪ Three unipolar limb leads: aV_R, aV_L, and aV_F
▪ Record electrical activity in the heart's frontal plane, providing a view through the middle of the heart from top to bottom

The precordial leads

▪ Six unipolar precordial (chest) leads: V_1 through V_6
▪ Record electrical activity in the heart's horizontal plane, providing a transverse view through the middle of the heart, dividing it into upper and lower portions

Electrical axis

▪ Measurement of the electrical impulses flowing through the heart
▪ Normal axis downward and to the left
▪ Direction of electrical activity swings away from areas of damage or necrosis and toward areas of hypertrophy

Placing the leads

▪ Bipolar and unipolar limb leads: electrodes on both arms and the left leg, ground on right leg
– V_1: Over fourth intercostal space at right sternal border
– V_2: Over fourth intercostal space at left sternal border
– V_3: Midway between leads V_2 and V_4
– V_4: Over fifth intercostal space at left midclavicular line
– V_5: Over fifth intercostal space at left anterior axillary line
– V_6: Over fifth intercostal space at left midaxillary line

VIEWS OF THE HEART WALLS

▪ Lead I: Lateral wall
▪ Lead II: Inferior wall
▪ Lead III: Inferior wall
▪ Lead aV_R: No specific view
▪ Lead aV_L: Lateral wall
▪ Lead aV_F: Inferior wall
▪ Lead V_1: Septal wall
▪ Lead V_2: Septal wall
▪ Lead V_3: Anterior wall
▪ Lead V_4: Anterior wall
▪ Lead V_5: Lateral wall
▪ Lead V_6: Lateral wall

OTHER LEAD PLACEMENTS

▪ Posterior leads: V_7, V_8, and V_9 are placed opposite V_4, V_5, and V_6 on the left side of the back to view posterior surface of the heart
– V_7: Over fifth intercostal space at posterior axillary line
– V_8: Midway between leads V_8 and V_9
– V_9: Over fifth intercostal space at paraspinal line
▪ Right chest leads: placed on right chest in mirror image of standard precordial leads to view right ventricle
– V_{1R}: Over fourth intercostal space at left sternal border
– V_{2R}: Over fourth intercostal space at right sternal border
– V_{3R}: Midway between leads V_{2R} and V_{4R}
– V_{4R}: Over fifth intercostal space at right midclavicular line
– V_{5R}: Over fifth intercostal space at right anterior axillary line
– V_{6R}: Over fifth intercostal space at right midaxillary line

Types of ECGs

▪ Multichannel ECG: All electrodes attached at one time to provide simultaneous views of all leads
▪ Signal-averaged ECG: Use of computer to identify late electrical potentials from three specialized leads over hundreds of beats; identifies patients at risk for sudden cardiac death from ventricular tachycardia

■ Batter's box

Before jumping into the workout, let's review a few key concepts. Fill in the blanks with the appropriate words.

Elementary leads

The 12-lead ECG is a diagnostic test that helps identify _____
1

conditions, especially _____ and acute _____ . It gives a
2   3

more complete view of the heart's electrical activity than a _____ and
4

can be used to assess left _____ function.
5

    A 12-lead ECG must be viewed alongside other clinical evidence. Always

correlate the patient's ECG results with his _____ ,
6

_____ assessment findings, _____ results, and
7   8

_____ regimen.
9

Remember, too, that an ECG can be done in a variety of ways, including over a

_____ line. _____ monitoring, in fact, has become
10   11

increasingly important as a tool for assessing patients at _____ or in
12

other nonclinical settings.

Lead activity

The 12-lead ECG records the heart's electrical activity using a series of

_____ placed on the patient's _____ and
13   14

_____ wall. The 12 leads include three _____ limb
15   16

leads, three _____ augmented limb leads, and six unipolar
17

_____ , or chest, leads. These leads provide 12 different
18

_____ of the heart's electrical activity.
19

Options

angina
bipolar
chest
electrodes
extremities
history
home
laboratory
medication
myocardial infarction
pathologic
physical
precordial
rhythm strip
telephone
transtelephonic
unipolar
ventricular
views

■■
■ Strike out

Some of the statements below about 12-lead ECGs are incorrect. Cross out the incorrect statements.

1. Waveforms obtained from each lead vary depending on the location of the lead in relation to the wave of depolarization passing through the epicardium.

2. The six limb leads record electrical activity in the heart's horizontal plane.

3. The six precordial leads record electrical activity from either a superior or an inferior approach.

4. The three unipolar augmented leads are aV_R, aV_L, and aV_F.

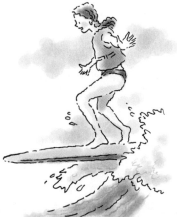

You're at a pivotal point! Try not to wipe out on this one.

■■
■ Cross-training

Complete this crossword puzzle using the clues below.

Across

3. A measurement of electrical impulses flowing through the heart

5. Another term for electrical axis: mean _____ vector

7. In a normal axis, the movement of the impulses is _____ and to the left

8. One of the views used to record electrical activity in the heart's horizontal plane

9. Plane that provides a view through the middle of the heart from top to bottom

Down

1. A heart condition in which a 12-lead ECG may be used

2. The heart's horizontal plane provides a _____ view

4. In a damaged heart, the direction of electrical activity swings toward areas of _____

6. Impulses travel through the heart generating small electrical forces called instantaneous _____

■ Finish line

This illustration shows the direction of each lead in a 12-lead ECG relative to the wave of depolarization.
Can you label all of the leads?

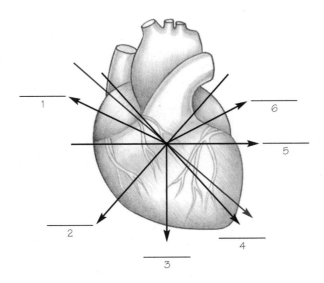

■ Match point

How much do you know about standard and augmented limb leads? See if you can match each of the following leads with its appropriate type of lead and view of the heart.

1. I _____   A. Bipolar lead; inferior wall

2. II or III _____   B. Unipolar lead; inferior wall

3. aV$_R$ _____   C. Unipolar lead; no specific view

4. aV$_L$ _____   D. Bipolar lead; lateral wall

5. aV$_F$ _____   E. Unipolar lead; lateral wall

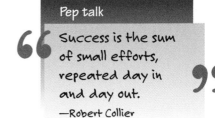

Pep talk

Success is the sum of small efforts, repeated day in and day out.

—Robert Collier

Finish line

Use this illustration to label the precordial leads and the area of the heart revealed by each.

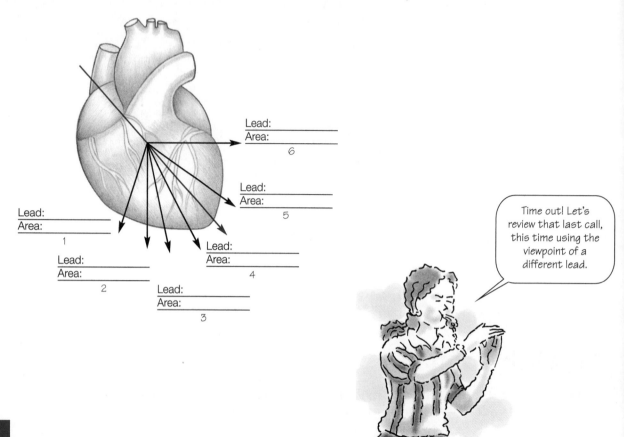

Lead: _____
Area: _____
6

Lead: _____
Area: _____
5

Lead: _____
Area: _____
1

Lead: _____
Area: _____
2

Lead: _____
Area: _____
3

Lead: _____
Area: _____
4

Time out! Let's review that last call, this time using the viewpoint of a different lead.

Hit or miss

Some of the following statements about 12-lead ECGs are true; the others are false. Label each one accordingly.

_____ 1. Obtaining a 12-lead ECG usually takes about 30 minutes.

_____ 2. Inaccurate placement of an electrode by greater than ⅜″ from its standardized position may lead to inaccurate waveforms.

_____ 3. A firm, muscular area is ideal for electrode placement.

_____ 4. In preparation of obtaining an ECG, the patient should lie supine in the center of the bed with his arms at his sides.

■■ Match point

Test your knowledge of left precordial lead placement by matching each of the precordial leads below with its correct electrode position.

1. V_1 _____   A. Fifth intercostal space at the left anterior axillary line

2. V_2 _____   B. Fifth intercostal space at the left midaxillary line

3. V_3 _____   C. Fourth intercostal space at the left sternal border

4. V_4 _____   D. Fourth intercostal space at the right sternal border

5. V_5 _____   E. Fifth intercostal space at the left midclavicular line

6. V_6 _____   F. Midway between the fourth intercostal space, left sternal border and the fifth intercostal space, left midclavicular line

■■ Finish line

Test your knowledge of right precordial lead placement by labeling each lead on the following illustration.

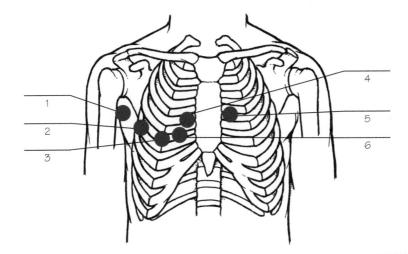

■■
■ Finish line

Test your knowledge of posterior lead placement by labeling each lead on the following illustration.

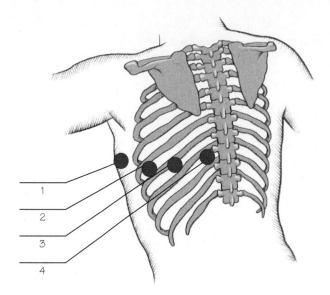

1. _____
2. _____
3. _____
4. _____

■■
■ Mind sprints

Go the distance by listing in 1 minute five reasons that a 12-lead ECG may be ordered for a patient.

1. _____

2. _____

3. _____

4. _____

5. _____

■■
■ Strike out

Some of the statements below are incorrect. Cross out the incorrect statements.

1. Three posterior leads may be added to the 12-lead ECG: leads V_7, V_8, and V_9.

2. Leads V_{7R}, V_{8R}, and V_{9R} provide information on the right anterior area of the heart.

3. A doctor may order a right chest lead ECG for a patient with an inferior wall MI.

4. A right chest lead ECG may be ordered to identify damage to the right atria.

■■
■ Jumble gym

Unscramble the words to uncover terms related to obtaining a 12-lead ECG. Then use the circled letters to answer the question below.

Question: A standard 12-lead ECG evaluates the function of what area of the heart?

1. Records activity in the heart's frontal plane

   B L I M   D E A L ◯ _ _ _ _◯ _ _

2. Usual chest leads can't "see" this area of the heart

   O T O P R I E S R _ _ _◯ _ _◯ _ _

3. Where precordial leads are placed

   I L A T N S C T E O R   C P S A E

   _◯ _ _ _ _ _ _◯ _ _   _ _ _ _◯

4. Name for chest leads

   D R E L I R P O C A _ _ _◯ _ _ _ _ _◯

5. Placed on a patient's extremities and chest wall

   D T E E S L C O R E _ _ _ _ _◯ _ _◯ _

6. Varies according to lead location

   F M A W R V E O _ _◯ _◯ _ _ _

Answer: _ _ _ _   _ _ _ _ _ _ _ _ _

> Learning to obtain a 12-lead ECG is like walking up a flight of stairs. You'll get there if you take it one step at a time.

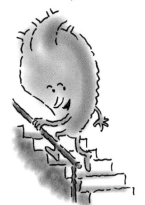

You make the call

Proper lead placement is critical for accurate recording of cardiac rhythms. Using the diagrams below, show the electrode placement for the six limb leads by inserting dots where the leads would be placed. Label the negative and positive poles, as well as the ground when appropriate. Finally, draw a line showing the angle of the view of the heart obtained by each lead.

Lead I

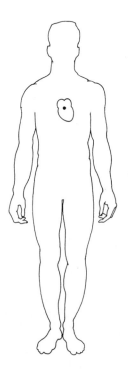

Lead II

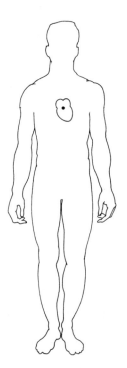

Lead III

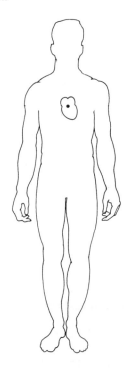

Lead aV_R

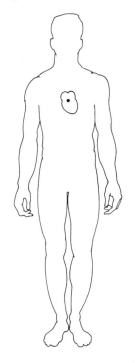

Lead aV_L

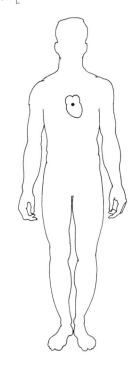

Lead aV_F

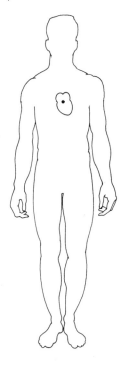

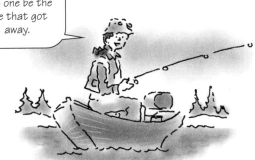

Cross-training

Complete this crossword puzzle using the clues below.

Across

2. Lead _____ separate the lead recordings on the paper

3. The patient shouldn't _____ during the ECG recording to prevent distortion of the tracing

6. If a patient has high _____ complexes, the marks on the ECG recording will be half as high

8. Standardization marks on an ECG recording are _____ squares high

9. Type of outlet an ECG machine should be plugged into

Down

1. ECGs are this kind of document

2. Type of ECG machine: _____ recorder

4. The ECG _____ speed selector should be set to 25 mm/second

5. Rate that appears at the top of the patient's ECG printout

7. Number of electrodes placed at a time for a single-channel recorder

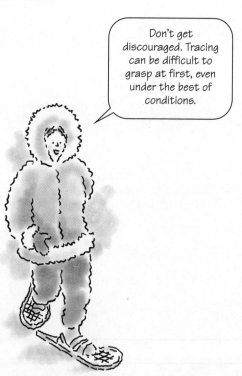

Don't get discouraged. Tracing can be difficult to grasp at first, even under the best of conditions.

Starting lineup

Test your ECG machine knowledge. Put the following steps in the order they should be performed.

Place one or all of the electrodes on the patient's chest, based on the type of machine you're using.	1.
Set the ECG paper speed selector and calibrate the machine according to the manufacturer's instructions.	2.
Remove the electrodes from the patient.	3.
Plug in the ECG machine.	4.
Instruct the patient to relax, lie still, and breathe normally.	5.
Observe the quality of the tracing.	6.
Press the AUTO button and record the ECG.	7.
Make sure all leads are securely attached.	8.

Hit or miss

Some of the following statements about signal-averaged ECGs are true; the others are false. Label each one accordingly.

_____ 1. A signal-averaged ECG identifies patients at risk for sudden death from type II second-degree AV block.

_____ 2. The machine averages signals to produce one representative QRS complex without artifacts.

_____ 3. A signal-averaged ECG is a surface ECG recording taken from two specialized leads for several hundred heartbeats.

_____ 4. Electrical potentials are tiny impulses that follow normal repolarization.

■ Finish line

Label the electrodes for a signal-averaged ECG.

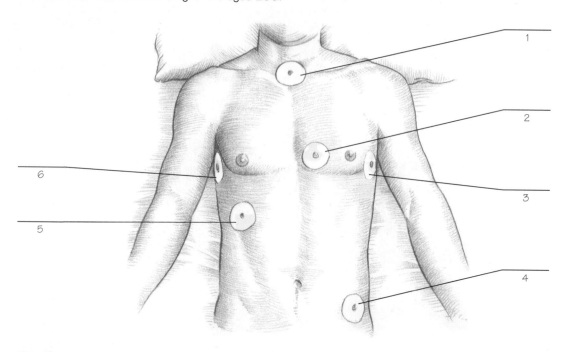

■ Match point

Match each of the signal-averaged electrodes below with its correct placement.

1. Z– _____   A. Left iliac crest

2. Y– _____   B. Back

3. G _____   C. Superior aspect of the manubrium of the sternum

4. Y+ _____   D. Lower right at eighth rib

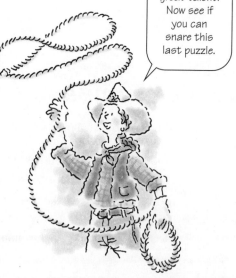

You've got great talent! Now see if you can snare this last puzzle.

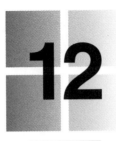

Interpreting a 12-lead ECG

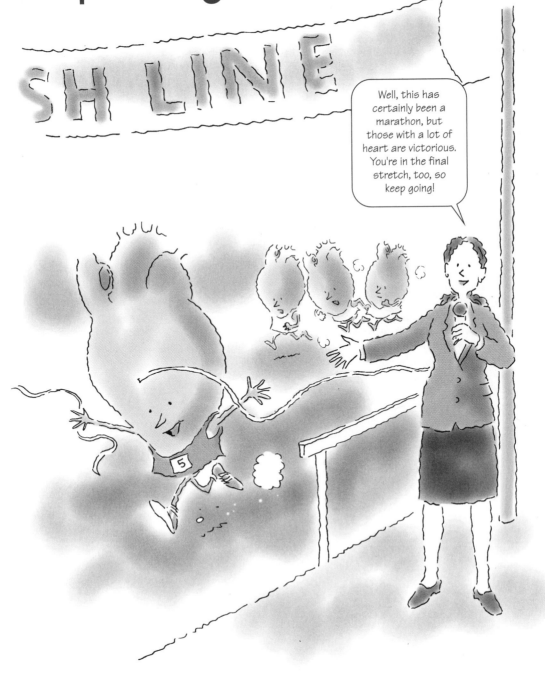

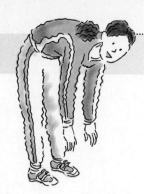

Interpreting a 12-lead ECG review

Looking at the waves

- P waves: Upright; possibly inverted in lead aV_R or biphasic or inverted in leads III, aV_L, and V_1
- PR intervals: Always constant, like QRS-complex durations
- QRS-complex deflections: Variable in different leads
- Q waves: Possibly pathologic; has a duration of less than 0.4 second when normal
- T wave: Slightly rounded and upright; normal deflection upward in leads I, II, and V_3 through V_6; inverted in lead III, aV_R, aV_F, aV_L, and V_1; should not be tall, peaked, or notched
- ST segments: should be isoelectric or have minimal deviation

Electrical axis

- Average direction of the heart's electrical activity during ventricular depolarization

METHODS OF DETERMINING AXIS

- Quadrant method: Determines main deflection of QRS complex in leads I and aV_F
- Degree method: Identifies axis by degrees on the hexaxial system
- Examination of the waveforms from the six frontal leads: I, II, III, aV_R, aV_L, and aV_F
- Normal axis: Between 0 and +90 degrees
- Left axis deviation: Between 0 and –90 degrees
- Right axis deviation: Between +90 and +180 degrees
- Extreme axis deviation: Between –180 and –90 degrees

Disorders affecting 12-lead ECGs

Angina

- Possible ECG changes: peaked or flattened T wave, T-wave inversion, and ST-segment depression with or without T-wave inversion

Bundle-branch block

- QRS complex: Width increases to greater than 0.12 second with bundle-branch block
- Lead V_1 (to right of heart) and V_6 (to left of heart): Used to determine whether block is in right or left bundle
- Right bundle-branch block: QRS complex has rsR′ pattern and T-wave inversion in lead V_1 and widened S wave and upright T wave in lead V_6
- Left bundle-branch block: Wide S wave (which may be preceded by a Q wave or small R wave) and small positive T wave in lead V_1; tall, notched R wave or slurred R wave and T-wave inversion in lead V_6

MI

- Three pathologic changes on ECG—ischemia, injury, and infarction

PATHOLOGIC ECG CHANGES

- Zone of ischemia: T-wave inversion
- Zone of injury: ST-segment elevation
- Zone of infarction: Pathologic Q wave in transmural myocardial infarction (MI)

LOCATING THE MI

- Anterior wall: Leads V_2 to V_4; involves LAD artery
- Anteroseptal wall: Leads V_1 to V_4; involves LAD artery
- Inferior wall: Leads II, III, aV_F; involves right coronary artery
- Lateral wall: Leads I, aV_L, V_5, V_6; involves left circumflex artery
- Posterior wall: Leads V_7, V_8, V_9; involves right coronary or left circumflex arteries
- Right ventricular wall: Leads V_{4R}, V_{5R}, V_{6R}; involves right coronary artery

■■
■ Starting lineup

Test your knowledge of interpreting 12-lead ECGs. Put the following steps in the order they should be performed.

Scan limb leads I, II, and III.	1.
Determine the electrical axis.	2.
Examine limb leads I, II, and III.	3.
Locate the lead markers on the waveform.	4.
Examine the R wave in the precordial leads.	5.
Check the standardization markings to make sure all leads were recorded with the ECG machine's amplitude at the same setting.	6.
Examine the S wave.	7.
Assess the heart rate and rhythm.	8.
Check the ECG tracing to see if it's technically correct. Make sure the baseline is free from electrical interference and drift.	9.
Examine limb leads aV_L, aV_F, and aV_R.	10.

You're off to a running start! Keep up the good work!

■■
■ Cross-training

Complete this crossword puzzle using the clues below.

Across

1. T waves may appear this way in lead III

2. From leads V_1 to V_6, the S wave gets smaller until it finally _____

4. R waves in lead II should be _____ than in lead I

7. Reference system created from imaginary lines drawn from each lead and intersecting at the center of the heart

10. The T wave normally deflects _____ in leads I, II, and V_3 through V_6

11. Characteristic of normal ST segments

12. Dominant R waves in the chest leads and upright T waves are normal findings in these patients

Down

1. This may be indicated with excessively tall, flat, or inverted T waves

3. Q wave that generally has a duration of less than 0.04 second

5. The average direction of the heart's electrical activity during ventricular depolarization: electrical _____

6. Pathological Q waves indicate myocardial _____

8. Leads sense the _____ of the heart's electrical activity

9. Leads _____ an injured area show ST-segment elevation

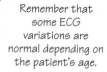

Remember that some ECG variations are normal depending on the patient's age.

■■
■ Hit or miss

Some of the following statements about the quadrant method for determining electrical axis are true; the others are false. Label each one accordingly.

_____ 1. The quadrant method is the more precise axis calculation.

_____ 2. If lead I is upright and lead aV_F points down, right axis deviation exists.

_____ 3. In the quadrant method, lead I indicates whether the impulses are right or left.

_____ 4. If the QRS-complex deflection is negative or downward in both leads, the electrical axis is normal.

■■
■ Starting lineup

The following steps should be taken when using the degree method of axis calculation. Put the steps in order.

Review all six leads.

Plot the information on the hexaxial diagram to determine the direction of the electrical axis.

Use the hexaxial diagram to identify the lead perpendicular to this lead.

Examine the perpendicular lead's QRS complex.

Identify the lead that contains either the smallest QRS complex or the complex with an equal deflection above and below the baseline.

1.

2.

3.

4.

5.

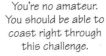
You're no amateur. You should be able to coast right through this challenge.

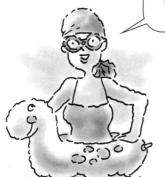

■■ You make the call
■

Using the illustrations below as a guide, explain the steps involved in determining axis deviation by the degree method.

Step 1

_____

_____

_____

_____

Lead I	Lead II	Lead III	Lead aV$_R$	Lead aV$_L$	Lead aV$_F$
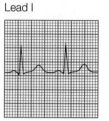	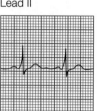	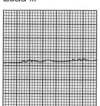	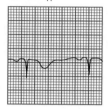	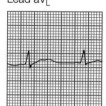	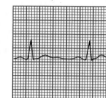

Step 2

_____

_____

_____

_____

_____

_____

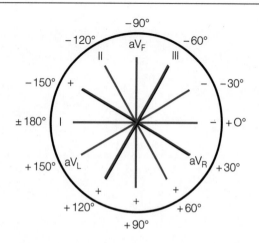

Step 3

_____

_____

_____

_____

_____

_____

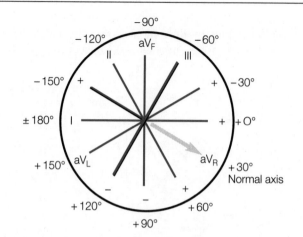

Team up

How well do you know the causes of axis deviation? In the list below, label the conditions that can cause left axis deviation with an "L" and label those that can cause right axis deviation with an "R."

_____ 1. Lateral wall MI

_____ 2. Left bundle-branch block

_____ 3. Emphysema

_____ 4. Aging

_____ 5. Wolff-Parkinson-White syndrome

_____ 6. Inferior wall myocardial infarction

_____ 7. Left posterior hemiblock

Strike out

Some of the statements below about angina are incorrect. Cross out the incorrect statements.

1. Angina shows ischemic changes on the ECG only during the angina attack.

2. Drugs used to treat angina include quinidine, morphine sulfate, and angiotensin-converting enzyme.

3. Stable angina is unpredictable and worsens over time.

4. In angina, the myocardium demands more oxygen than the coronary arteries can deliver.

5. If an angina episode lasts close to 10 minutes, it's more likely that the pain is from an MI.

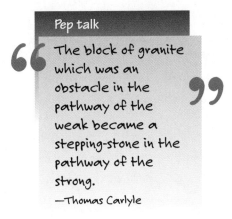

Pep talk

The block of granite which was an obstacle in the pathway of the weak became a stepping-stone in the pathway of the strong.

—Thomas Carlyle

■ Match point

Match each of the ECG changes associated with angina below to its appropriate illustration.

1. ST-segment depression without T-wave inversion _____
2. T-wave inversion _____
3. Flattened T wave _____
4. ST-segment depression with T-wave inversion _____
5. Peaked T wave _____

Practice your technique with this ECG brain-teaser.

A.

B.

C.

D.

E.

■ Team up

How well can you differentiate right bundle-branch block from left bundle-branch block? In the list below, label the characteristics of RBBB with an "R" and the characteristics of LBBB with an "L."

_____ 1. The initial impulse activates the interventricular septum from left to right (as in normal activation).

_____ 2. The initial impulse travels down the right bundle branch and activates the interventricular septum from right to left (the opposite of normal activation).

_____ 3. When this block occurs along with an anterior wall MI, it usually signals complete heart block.

_____ 4. Lead V_1 shows a small R wave followed by an S wave, a tall R wave, and a negative T wave.

_____ 5. Lead V_1 shows a wide S wave (possibly preceded by a Q wave or a small R wave) and a positive T wave.

_____ 6. Lead V_6 shows no initial Q wave and a tall, notched R wave or a slurred one.

_____ 7. In lead V_6, a small Q wave is followed by a tall R wave and a broad S wave.

_____ 8. In lead V_6, the T wave is positive.

_____ 9. In lead V_6, the T wave is negative.

Cross-training

Complete this crossword puzzle using the clues below.

Across

3. A second R wave that occurs after an initial R wave is called R _____

7. In a bundle-branch block, either the left or right bundle branch fails to conduct _____

9. Bundle-branch block that occurs farther down the left bundle, in the posterior or anterior fasciculus

10. Characteristic of QRS complex in bundle-branch block

13. The "A" in CAD

14. Form of angina that's treated as a medical emergency

15. ECG changes from angina are _____

Down

1. In LBBB, the ventricles are activated _____ , not simultaneously

2. Type of T wave produced in lead I in a LBBB

4. A block that develops as the heart rate increases is called a _____-related RBBB

5. In lead V_6 of LBBB, the R wave appears tall and notched, or it may be _____

6. Aortic _____ is one cause of LBBB

8. Type of bundle-branch block that may occur without cardiac disease

11. Type of bundle-branch block that never occurs normally

12. In RBBB, QRS complexes sometimes resemble _____ ears

Keep moving. It's a simple way to improve blood flow to your heart.

■ You make the call

Identify the condition that the following 12-lead ECG indicates. Then describe the characteristic changes seen in the rhythm strips.

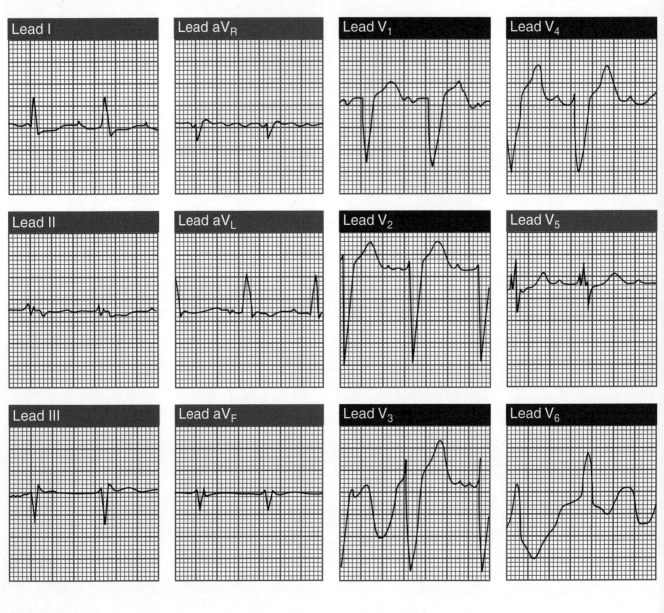

Lead I	Lead aV_R	Lead V_1	Lead V_4
Lead II	Lead aV_L	Lead V_2	Lead V_5
Lead III	Lead aV_F	Lead V_3	Lead V_6

Answer: _____

_____

_____

_____

■ Jumble gym

Use the clues below to help you unscramble terms related to MI. Then use the circled letters to answer the question below.

Question: If MI symptoms persist for more than 6 hours, little can be done to prevent what?

1. MI usually occurs here

   T E F L   L C E E T V I N R   _ O _ _   _ _ O _ _ _ _ _ _

2. Results when tissue is deprived of an oxygen-rich blood supply

   M I S C A H E I   _ O _ _ _ _ O _

3. A common symptom of MI

   C T S H E   I P A N   O _ _ O _   _ _ _ _

4. Pathologic changes reflected on an ECG

   F T I I N A C R O N   _ _ _ _ O _ _ _ O _

Answer: _ _ _ _ _ _ _ _

■ Hit or miss

Some of the following statements about MI are true; the others are false. Label each one accordingly.

_____ 1. An area of myocardial necrosis is called injury.

_____ 2. Pathologic Q waves reflect poor depolarization

_____ 3. An elevated ST segment indicates that myocardial injury is occurring.

_____ 4. Inverted T waves return to baseline within a few days to 2 weeks.

_____ 5. Treatment for an MI includes decreasing cardiac workload and increasing oxygen supply to the myocardium.

■ Match point

The lead used to monitor a patient with an MI depends on the area of infarction. Match each type of MI in the list below on the left with the most appropriate lead for ongoing monitoring on the right.

1. Lateral wall MI _____
2. Anterior wall MI _____
3. Inferior wall MI _____
4. Septal wall MI _____

A. V_6 or MCL_6

B. Lead II

C. V_1 or MCL_1

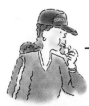

Coaching session
Locating myocardial damage

After you've noted characteristic lead changes of an acute myocardial infarction, use this chart to identify the areas of damage. Match the lead changes in the second column with the affected wall in the first column and the artery involved in the third column. Column four shows reciprocal lead changes.

Wall affected	Leads	Artery involved	Reciprocal changes
Anterior	V_2 to V_4	Left coronary artery, left anterior descending (LAD) artery	II, III, aV_F
Anterolateral	I, aV_L, V_3 to V_6	LAD artery, circumflex artery	II, III, aV_F
Anteroseptal	V_1 to V_4	LAD artery	None
Inferior (diaphragmatic)	II, III, aV_F	Right coronary artery	I, aV_L
Lateral	I, aV_L, V_5, V_6	Circumflex artery, branch of left coronary artery	II, III, aV_F
Posterior	V_8, V_9	Right coronary artery, circumflex artery	V_1 to V_4
Right ventricular	V_{4R}, V_{5R}, V_{6R}	Right coronary artery	None

■ Finish line

Fill in the area of the heart with the appropriate leads that monitor damage to those areas.

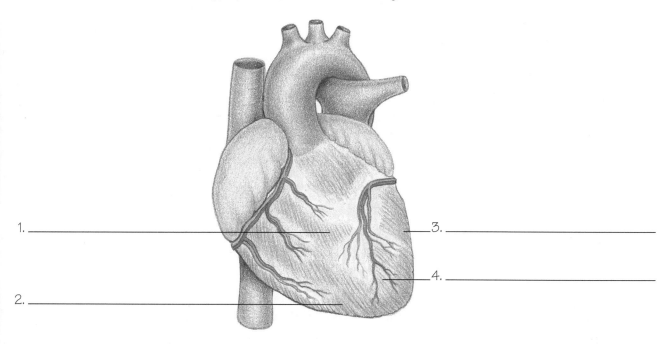

1. _____

2. _____

3. _____

4. _____

■ Fair or foul?

Can you identify the treatments that are indicated for improving blood flow to the heart of a patient who has had an MI? Circle the characteristics that are correct.

1. Stent placement

2. Synchronized cardioversion

3. Intra-aortic balloon pump

4. Implantable cardioverter-defibrillator

5. Coronary artery bypass graft

6. Catheter ablation

7. Atherectomy

■ Strike out

Some of the statements below about MI are incorrect. Cross out the incorrect statements.

1. The LAD artery supplies blood to the ventricular septum so a septal wall MI often accompanies an anterior wall MI.

2. A right ventricular MI is also called a diaphragmatic MI.

3. 40% of all patients with an inferior wall MI also suffer a right ventricular MI.

4. A lateral wall MI usually accompanies an anterior and posterior wall MI.

5. Identifying an anterior wall MI is difficult without information from the right precordial leads.

■ Match point

Match each of the following types of MI with its corresponding characteristics.

1. Right ventricular MI _____

2. Posterior wall MI _____

3. Anterior wall MI _____

4. Inferior wall MI _____

5. Septal wall MI _____

A. ECG changes include a disappearing R wave, rising ST segment, and an inverted T wave in leads V_1 and V_2

B. Caused by occlusion of the right coronary artery

C. Can lead to right-sided heart failure or right-sided block

D. ECG changes include tall R waves, ST-segment depression, and upright T waves in leads V_1 and V_2

E. Complications of this MI include varying second–degree blocks, bundle-branch blocks, ventricular irritability, and left-sided heart failure

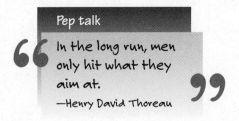

Pep talk

In the long run, men only hit what they aim at.

—Henry David Thoreau

You make the call

Identify the condition that the following 12-lead ECG indicates. Then describe the characteristic changes seen in the rhythm strips.

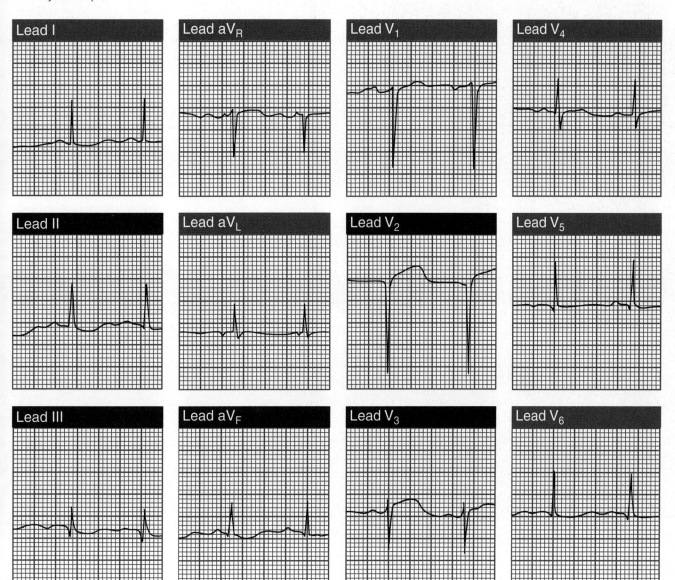

Answer: _____

_____

_____

_____

■ You make the call

Identify the condition that the following 12-lead ECG indicates. Then describe the characteristic changes seen in the rhythm strips.

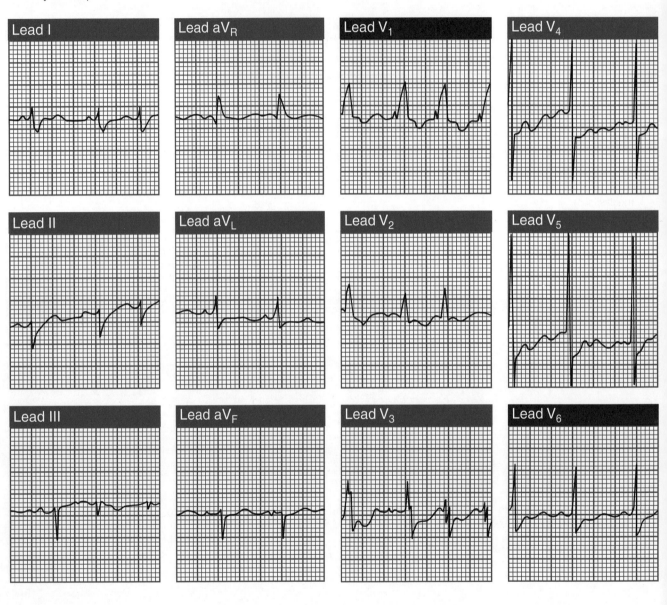

Answer: _____

_____

_____

_____

■ Answers

■ Chapter 1

■ Page 3
Batter's box

1. mediastinum; 2. lungs; 3. second; 4. left; 5. epicardium; 6. epithelial; 7. myocardium; 8. largest; 9. endocardium; 10. endothelial; 11. four; 12. atria; 13. ventricles; 14. valves; 15. atrioventricular; 16. semilunar; 17. vena cavae; 18. atrium; 19. tricuspid valve; 20. right; 21. lungs; 22. aorta

■ Page 4
Finish line

1. Endocardium
2. Myocardium
3. Epicardium (visceral layer of serous pericardium)
4. Parietal layer of serous pericardium
5. Fibrous pericardium

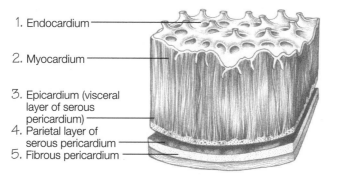

Strike out

1. ~~The serous pericardium has 3 layers~~. The serous pericardium, the thin, smooth, inner portions of the pericardium, has two layers: the parietal layer, which lines the inside of the fibrous pericardium, and the visceral layer, which adheres to the surface of the heart.
4. ~~The parietal layer adheres to the surface of the heart~~. The visceral layer of the pericardium adheres to the surface of the heart.

■ Page 5

Cross-training

```
                    ¹A O ²R T I C
                        E
                        G
                        U      ³M
⁴T H I C K N E S ⁵S     R       I
 W                 E     G       T
 O       ⁶S E P T U M    I       R
                   I     T       A
                  ⁷L E A F L E ⁸T S
                   U     T       R
                   N     I       I
         ⁹C        A     O       C
        ¹⁰M U R M U R    N       U
          S                     S
          P                     P
          S                     I
        ¹¹O X Y G E N A T E D
```

■ Page 6

Finish line

1. Superior vena cava 2. Branches of right pulmonary artery 3. Right atrium 4. Right pulmonary veins 5. Tricuspid valve 6. Chordae tendineae 7. Interventricular septum 8. Right ventricle 9. Papillary muscle 10. Inferior vena cava 11. Descending aorta 12. Aortic arch 13. Pulmonic valve 14. Branches of left pulmonary artery 15. Left atrium 16. Left pulmonary veins 17. Mitral valve 18. Myocardium 19. Aortic valve 20. Left ventricle

Jumble gym

1. Ventricles 2. Venae cavae 3. Coronary sinus 4. Cusps

Answer: Pressure

■ Page 7

You make the call

1. Superior vena cava 2. Right atrium 3. Tricuspid valve; right ventricle 4. Pulmonic valve; pulmonary arteries 5. Pulmonary veins; left atrium 6. Mitral valve; left ventricle 7. Aortic valve; aorta

■ Page 8

You make the call

1. Isovolumetric ventricular contraction—Tension in the ventricles increases in response to ventricular depolarization. The mitral and tricuspid valves close, and the pulmonic and aortic valves stay closed during the entire phase.
2. Ventricular ejection—When ventricular pressure exceeds aortic and pulmonary arterial pressures (80 mm Hg), the aortic and pulmonic valves open and the ventricles eject 70% of the blood.
3. Isovolumetric relaxation—When ventricular pressure falls below pressure in the aorta and pulmonary artery, the aortic and pulmonic valves close (all valves are closed during this phase). Atrial diastole occurs as blood fills the atria.
4. Ventricular filling—Atrial pressure exceeds ventricular pressure, which causes the mitral and tricuspid valves to open. Blood then flows passively into the ventricles. About 70% of ventricular filling takes place during this phase.
5. Atrial systole—Also known as *atrial kick,* atrial systole supplies the ventricles with the remaining 30% of the blood for each heartbeat.

■ Page 9

Hit or miss

1. True.
2. False. Cardiac output is the amount of blood the heart pumps in 1 minute.
3. True.
4. True.
5. False. Preload refers to passive stretching exerted by blood on the ventricular muscles at the end of diastole.

Jumble gym

1. **Stroke volume** 2. **Cardiac cycle** 3. **Atrial systole** 4. **Afterload**

Answer: Diastole

■ Page 10

You make the call

- *Phase 0:* Rapid depolarization—Sodium moves rapidly into the cell; calcium moves slowly into the cell.
- *Phase 1:* Early repolarization—Sodium channels close.
- *Phase 2:* Plateau phase—Calcium continues to flow in; potassium flows out of the cell.
- *Phase 3:* Rapid repolarization—Calcium channels close; potassium flows out rapidly.
- *Phase 4:* Resting phase—Active transport through the sodium-potassium pump begins restoring potassium to the inside of the cell and sodium to the outside, the cell membrane becomes impermeable to sodium, and potassium may move out of the cell.

Match point

1. B, 2. D, 3. A, 4. E, 5. C

■ Page 11

Strike out

1. ~~The parasympathetic nervous system is the heart's accelerator.~~ The parasympathetic nervous system serves as the heart's brakes. The vagus nerve of this system carries impulses that slow heart rate and the conduction of impulses through the AV node and ventricles.
3. ~~Acetylcholine increases heart rate, automaticity, atrioventricular conduction, and contractility.~~ Acetylcholine, a chemical that's released when parasympathetic nervous system is stimulated, slows the heart rate.

Hit or miss

1. True.
2. False. Preload is the passive stretching exerted by blood on the ventricular muscle at the end of diastole.
3. False. Starling's law says that the more the cardiac muscles stretch in diastole, the more forcefully they contract in systole.
4. True.

■ **Page 12**

Match point

1. C, 2. B, 3. D, 4. A

■ **Page 13**

Jumble gym

1. Polarized 2. Impulse 3. Action potential curve 4. Voltage
Answer: Resting

Starting lineup

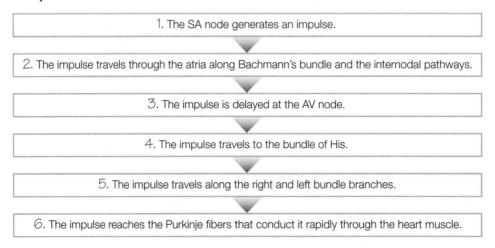

1. The SA node generates an impulse.

2. The impulse travels through the atria along Bachmann's bundle and the internodal pathways.

3. The impulse is delayed at the AV node.

4. The impulse travels to the bundle of His.

5. The impulse travels along the right and left bundle branches.

6. The impulse reaches the Purkinje fibers that conduct it rapidly through the heart muscle.

■ **Page 14**

Finish line

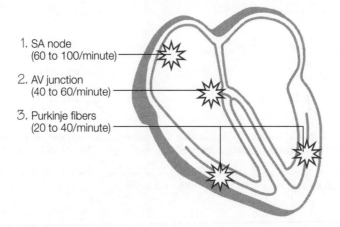

1. SA node
(60 to 100/minute)

2. AV junction
(40 to 60/minute)

3. Purkinje fibers
(20 to 40/minute)

Train your brain

Answer: Purkinje fibers can serve as a pacemaker if the bundle of His becomes blocked.

Page 15

Strike out

2. ~~Early afterdepolarization can be caused by hypercalcemia.~~ Early afterdepolarization, which occurs before a cell is fully repolarized, can be caused by hypokalemia, slow pacing rates, or drug toxicity.

Match point

1. C, 2. A, 3. D, 4. B

Page 16

Cross-training

Page 17

Match point

1. B, 2. A, 3. C

Hit or miss

1. False. Automaticity is a special characteristic of pacemaker cells, not Purkinje fibers.
2. True.
3. False. Impulses that begin below the AV node can be transmitted backward toward the atria, not the ventricles.
4. True.
5. True.

■ Page 18

Odd man out

1. <u>Lungs</u>. The heart, blood vessels, and lymphatics are all components of the cardiovascular system. The lungs are not.
2. <u>Pericardium</u>. The epicardium, endocardium, and myocardium are layers of the heart wall. The pericardium is the sac that surrounds the heart.
3. <u>Mediastinum</u>. The atria and ventricles are the chambers of the heart. The mediastinum is the cavity between the lungs in which the heart is located.
4. <u>Pulmonic</u>. The bicuspid valve (also known as the *mitral valve*) and the tricuspid valve are AV valves; the pulmonic valve is a semilunar valve.
5. <u>Alveoli</u>. Arteries, venules, veins, arterioles, and capillaries are types of blood vessels. Alveoli are sacs in the terminal bronchioles of the lungs, in which carbon dioxide and oxygen exchange occurs.
6. <u>Intrinsic</u>. Systemic, coronary, and pulmonary are the three methods of circulation that carry blood throughout the body.

Circuit training

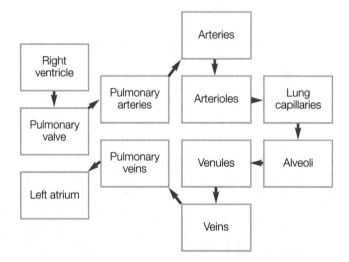

■ Chapter 2

■ Page 21

Batter's box

1. electrical; 2. tissue; 3. skin; 4. electrodes; 5. electrocardiogram; 6. waveforms; 7. depolarization; 8. repolarization; 9. cardiac; 10. contraction; 11. rhythm; 12. conduction; 13. baseline; 14. function; 15. leads; 16. planes; 17. positive; 18. negative; 19. frontal; 20. horizontal

■ Page 22

Match point

1. D, 2. C, 3. A, 4. B

You make the call

1. As current travels toward the negative pole, the waveform deflects mostly downward.
2. When current travels perpendicular to the lead, the waveform may be small or go in both directions (biphasic).
3. As current travels toward the positive pole, the waveform deflects mostly upward.

■ Page 23

Jumble gym

1. **I**soele**c**tric 2. **Wa**veform**s** 3. **B**aseline 4. **H**orizontal **p**lane

Answer: Biphasic

Strike out

2. ~~MCL stands for modified cardiac lead~~. MCL stands for "modified chest lead," not "modified cardiac lead."
3. ~~The six limb leads include leads V₁, V₂, V₃, V₄, V₅, and V₆~~. The six limb leads include I, II, III, augmented vector right (aV_R), augmented vector left (aV_L), and augmented vector foot (aV_F).

■ Page 24

Hit or miss

1. False. Leads I, II, and III require a negative and a positive electrode for monitoring, which makes these leads bipolar.
2. True.
3. True.
4. True.
5. False. Leads II and V_1 are the leads most commonly monitored simultaneously.

■ Page 25

Cross-training

		A(1)													
		U		B(2)			H(3)								
		G		I		D(4)	O	W	N	W	A	R	D		
U(5)		M		P			R								
P(6)	R	E	C	O	R	D	I	A	L						
W		N		L			Z								
A		T		A		C(7)	O	N	T	I	N	U	O	U	S
R		E		R			N								
D		D				S(8)	T	R	A	I	G	H	T(9)		
				D(10)			A						E		
V(11)	E	R	T	I	C	A	L						E		
				R									E		
				E									M		
				C									E		
	F(12)	O	O	T									T		
				I									R		
				O									Y		
			U(13)	N	I	P	O	L	A	R					

■ Page 26

Strike out

1. ~~Limited patient mobility is a drawback to telemetry monitoring.~~ Hardwire monitoring, not telemetry, limits the patient's mobility because the patient is tethered to a monitor by electrodes.
4. ~~Hardwire monitoring is generally used in step-down units and medical-surgical units.~~ Telemetry monitoring is generally used in step-down units and medical-surgical units where patients are permitted more activity.

Finish line

1. Lead I, 2. Right arm, 3. –, 4. –, 5. Lead II, 6. +, 7. Left leg, 8. Left arm, 9. +, 10. –, 11. Lead III, 12. +

■ Page 27

Match point

1. D, 2. C, 3. A, 4. B

■ Page 28

Hit or miss

1. True.
2. False. Lead aV_L shows electrical activity coming from the heart's lateral wall. Lead aV_R provides no specific view of the heart.
3. True.
4. False. Lead II tends to produce a positive, high-voltage deflection, resulting in tall P, R, and T waves.

Match point

1. D, 2. F, 3. A, 4. B, 5. E, 6. C

■ Page 29

Jumble gym

1. Unipolar 2. Electrical activity 3. Current 4. Precordial 5. Monitor

Answer: Ventricular

■ Page 30

Match point

1. E, 2. D, 3. B, 4. A, 5. C

■ Page 31

Strike out

1. ~~The three-electrode system is the only one that doesn't use a ground electrode.~~ The three-electrode system has one positive electrode, one negative electrode, and a ground.

Finish line

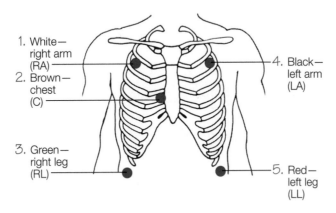

1. White—right arm (RA)
2. Brown—chest (C)
3. Green—right leg (RL)
4. Black—left arm (LA)
5. Red—left leg (LL)

■ Page 32

Starting lineup

1. Explain the electrode placement to the patient.

2. Choose electrode placement sites for the chosen lead.

3. If needed, clip dense hair closely at each site.

4. Prepare the patient's skin.

5. Apply the electrode.

Hit or miss

1. True.
2. False. Electrodes should be removed every 24 hours, not every 48 hours.
3. False. Electrodes should be placed over soft tissues or close to bone, not over bony prominences, thick muscles, or skin folds.
4. True.

■ Page 33

Cross-training

¹P	O	S	I	²T	I	O	N				
				R							
				A							
				C							
				I							
				N		³M				⁴T	
				⁵G	A	I	N			I	
						L				M	
			⁶A	M	P	L	I	T	U	D	E
			L			I					
			A			V					
			⁷R	E	C	O	R	D			
			M			L		⁸A			
			S			T		P			
			⁹B	A	S	E	L	I	N	E	
								C			
								A			
								L			

Jumble gym

1. **M**onitoring system 2. Cardiac **r**hythm 3. **H**eartbeat 4. Vertical ax**i**s

Answer: Arrhythmia

■ Page 34

Strike out

1. ~~Wandering baseline appears on the ECG as a baseline that's thick and unreadable.~~ A wandering baseline undulates, meaning that all waveforms are present but the baseline isn't stationary.
3. ~~Artifact interference is also called 60-cycle interference.~~ Electrical interference results in an ECG with a thick and unreadable baseline. Artifact is also called *waveform interference*.

Match point

1. C, 2. F, 3. A, 4. D, 5. B, 6. E

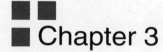

■ Chapter 3

■ Page 37

Match point

1. E, 2. C, 3. A, 4. F, 5. G, 6. D, 7. B

■ Page 38
Batter's box

1. electrical, 2. cardiac, 3. P, 4. Q, 5. R, 6. S, 7. T, 8. electrical, 9. impulses, 10. atria, 11. ventricles, 12. paper-and-pencil, 13. caliper, 14. intervals, 15. P, 16. R, 17. 1,500, 18. 10-times, 19. sequence

■ Page 39
Finish line

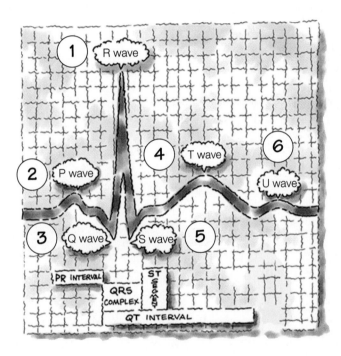

■ Page 40
Strike out

1. ~~Infants and children have faster heart rates than adults, producing long PR and QRS intervals~~. Infants and children have fast heart rates that produce short, not long, PR and QRS intervals.
2. ~~No P wave with the QRS complex may indicate hypercalcemia~~. No P wave with the QRS complex may indicate an atrial, junctional, or ventricular arrhythmia. The presence of a U wave or a shortened QT interval may indicate hypercalcemia
5. ~~In older adults, the QRS axis shifts to the right~~. In older adults, the QRS axis shifts to the left.

Hit or miss

1. False. Peaked, notched, or enlarged P waves may represent atrial hypertrophy or enlargement associated with chronic obstructive pulmonary disease, pulmonary emboli, valvular disease, or heart failure. Inverted P waves may indicate retrograde conduction from the atrioventricular junction toward the atria.
2. True.
3. True.
4. False. Deep, wide Q waves may represent myocardial infarction. A notched R wave may indicate a bundle-branch block.

■ Page 41

Jumble gym

1. Deflection 2. **B**iphasic 3. **A**mplitude 4. Con**d**uction

Answer: Absent

You make the call

1. The ST segment is depressed (5 mm or more below the baseline), possibly indicating myocardial ischemia or digoxin toxicity.
2. The ST segment is elevated (1 mm or more above the baseline), possibly indicating myocardial injury.

■ Page 42

Boxing match

2. depolarization, 3. amplitude, 4. deflection, 5. retrograde, 6. P wave

■ Page 43

Starting lineup

1. Determine the rhythm.
2. Determine the rate.
3. Evaluate the P wave.
4. Determine the duration of the PR interval.
5. Determine the duration of the QRS complex.
6. Evaluate the T waves.
7. Determine the duration of the QT interval.
8. Evaluate any other components.

Hit or miss

1. True.
2. False. To get an atrial rate using the sequence method, find a P wave that peaks on a heavy black line and assign the following numbers to the next six heavy black lines: 300, 150, 100, 75, 60, and 50.
3. False. The 1,500 method should be used if the heart rhythm is regular.
4. True.

Page 44

You make the call

- Rhythm: Atrial and ventricular rhythms are regular
- Rate: Atrial and ventricular rates are each 72 beats/minute
- P wave: Normal size and configuration
- PR interval: 0.20 second
- QRS complex: 0.10 second; normal size and configuration
- T wave: Normal configuration
- QT interval: 0.42 second
- Other: None
- Interpretation: Normal sinus rhythm

Page 45

Cross-training

Crossword solution:

- 1 Down: DURATION
- 2 Down: ELEVATED
- 3 Down: SHRT
- 4 Across: CONTRACTION
- 5 Down: CONDUCTION
- 6 Across: PULSE
- 7 Across: DEPOLARIZATION
- 8 Across: COUNTDOWN

Page 46

You make the call

- Rhythm: Atrial and ventricular rhythms are regular
- Rate: Atrial and ventricular rates are each 79 beats/minute
- P wave: Normal size and configuration
- PR interval: 0.12 second
- QRS complex: 0.08 second; normal size and configuration
- T wave: Normal configuration
- QT interval: 0.44 second
- Other: None
- Interpretation: Normal sinus rhythm

■ Page 47

Train your brain

Answer: The T wave shows ventricular recovery, or repolarization.

Strike out

2. ~~The slower the heart rate, the shorter the QT interval.~~ The faster the heart rate, the shorter the QT interval.
3. ~~Bumps in a T wave may indicate that a U wave is hidden in it.~~ Bumps in a T wave may indicate that a P wave is hidden in it, which means atrial depolarization has occurred.
6. ~~When documenting a QRS complex, uppercase letters should be used to indicate a wave with an amplitude greater than 3 mm.~~ Uppercase letters should be used to indicate a normal to high QRS amplitude (greater than 5 mm).

■ Page 48

Match point

1. D, 2. B, 3. C, 4. A

You make the call

1. The nurse is using the paper-and-pencil method to determine rhythm. She positions the straight edge of a piece of paper along the strip's baseline and uses a pencil to mark the peak of two consecutive R waves to measure the R-R interval.
2. The nurse is using the caliper method to determine rhythm. She places the ECG strip on a flat surface and positions the point of the caliper on the peak of the first R wave. Then she adjusts the caliper legs so the other point is on the peak of the next R wave. The distance between the points is the R-R interval.

■ Page 49

You make the call

- Rhythm: Atrial and ventricular rhythms are regular
- Rate: Atrial and ventricular rates are each 40 beats/minute
- P wave: Normal size and configuration
- PR interval: 0.20 second
- QRS complex: 0.10 second
- T wave: Peaked
- QT interval: 0.44 second
- Other: None

In case you were wondering, this rhythm represents sinus bradycardia, which will be discussed in more detail in chapter 4.

■ Page 50

Boxing match

2. baseline, 3. peak, 4. ventricular, 5. recovery, 6. rhythm, 7. irregular, 8. sequence

Hit or miss

1. True.
2. False. The sequence method uses the following numbers to establish heart rate: 300, 150, 100, 75, 60, and 50.
3. False. To determine atrial rhythm, measure the P-P intervals.
4. True.

Chapter 4

■ Page 53

Batter's box

1. pacemaker; 2. firing rate; 3. 60; 4. 100; 5. coronary; 6. circumflex; 7. autonomic; 8. vagus; 9. parasympathetic; 10. sympathetic; 11. vagus;12. sympathetic system; 13. arrhythmia; 14. SA node; 15. bradycardia; 16. 60; 17. regular; 18. tachycardia; 19. 100; 20. arrest; 21. atrium; 22. atrial standstill

■ Page 54

Hit or miss

1. False. During expiration, venous return decreases, which in turn increases vagal tone, slows the heart rate, and lengthens the P-P interval.
2. True.
3. True.
4. False. Sinus arrhythmia is easier to detect when the heart rate is slow.
5. True.

Jumble gym

1. Vagal tone 2. Expiration 3. Sinus node 4. Respiration

Answer: Digoxin

■ Page 55

You make the call

- Rhythm: Atrial and ventricular rhythms are irregular
- Rate: Atrial and ventricular rates are each 60 beats/minute
- P wave: Normal
- PR interval: 0.16 second
- QRS complex: 0.06 second
- T wave: Normal
- QT interval: 0.36 second
- Other: Phasic slowing and quickening
- Arrhythmia: Sinus arrhythmia

Strike out

1. ~~In sinus bradycardia, vagal stimulation decreases and sympathetic stimulation increases.~~ In sinus bradycardia, vagal stimulation increases and sympathetic stimulation decreases.
2. ~~Even if a patient is asymptomatic, sinus bradycardia is a serious condition that requires treatment.~~ Unless the patient shows symptoms of decreased cardiac output, no treatment is necessary.

■ Page 56

Starting lineup

| 1. Obtain and review a 12-lead ECG. |

⮟

| 2. Start an I.V. line, attach a monitor, and give I.V. fluids. |

⮟

| 3. Administer atropine, 0.5 to 1 mg. Repeat doses every 3 to 5 minutes to a total of 0.04 mg/kg. |

⮟

| 4. Perform transcutaneous pacing, if available. |

⮟

| 5. Administer dopamine, 5 to 20 mcg/kg/minute; administer epinephrine 2 to 10 mcg/minute. |

Fair or foul?

Causes of sinus bradycardia include:
1. Certain drugs, especially beta-adrenergic blockers, digoxin, and antiarrhythmics
2. Conditions producing excess vagal stimulation or decreased sympathetic stimulation
4. Noncardiac disorders, such as hyperkalemia, increased intracranial pressure, and glaucoma

■ Page 57

Match point

1. C, 2. B, 3. D, 4. A

Hit or miss

1. True.
2. False. An acute inferior wall MI usually causes sinus bradycardia not sinus tachycardia.
3. True.
4. True.

■ Page 58

You make the call

- Rhythm: Atrial and ventricular rhythms are regular
- Rate: Atrial and ventricular rates are each 48 beats/minute
- P wave: Normal
- PR interval: 0.16 second
- QRS complex: 0.08 second
- T wave: Normal
- QT interval: 0.50 second
- Other: None
- Arrhythmia: Sinus bradycardia

Page 59

Cross-training

```
 1I          2A  M  P  L  I  T  U  3D  E
  S                              I
  C                              A
  H       4C 5R  A  C  K 6L  E  S
  E          E        E  T
  M          G        V  O
  I          U        E  L
 7A  T  E  N  O  L  O  L  L     E
             A
        8E  X  E  R  C  I  S  E
```

Page 60

You make the call

- Rhythm: Atrial and ventricular rhythms are regular
- Rate: Atrial and ventricular rates are each 120 beats/minute
- P wave: Normal
- PR interval: 0.14 second
- QRS complex: 0.06 second
- T wave: Normal
- QT interval: 0.34 second
- Other: None
- Arrhythmia: Sinus tachycardia

Page 61

Strike out

1. ~~Atrial standstill is called sinus arrest when one or two beats aren't formed.~~ Atrial standstill is called sinus pause when one or two beats aren't formed. It is called sinus arrest when three or more beats aren't formed.
2. ~~With sinus arrest, the length of the pause is a multiple of the previous R-R intervals.~~ With sinus arrest, the length of the pause isn't a multiple of the previous R-R interval.

Power stretch

1. B, D
2. A, E
3. C, F
- Rhythm strip 1: Second-degree type II block
- Rhythm strip 2: Third-degree block
- Rhythm strip 3: Second-degree type I block

■ Page 62

You make the call

- Rhythm: Regular, except for the missing PQRST complexes
- Rate: Atrial and ventricular rates are each 40 beats/minute
- P wave: Normal; absent during pause
- PR interval: 0.20 second
- QRS complex: 0.08 second; absent during pause
- T wave: Normal; absent during pause
- QT interval: 0.40 second; absent during pause
- Other: None
- Arrhythmia: Sinus arrest

Jumble gym

1. Sinus pause 2. Arrhythmia 3. Cardiac output 4. Pacemaker

Answer: Syncope

■ Page 63

Match point

1. D, 2. B, 3. A, 4. C

Cross-training

■ Page 64
You make the call

- Rhythm: Atrial and ventricular rhythms are irregular
- Rate: Atrial is 60 beats/minute; ventricular rate is 70 beats/minute
- P wave: Configuration varies
- PR interval: Varies with rhythm
- QRS complex: 0.10 second
- T wave: Configuration varies
- QT interval: Varies with rhythm changes
- Other: None
- Arrhythmia: Sick sinus syndrome

Train your brain

Answer: In sinoatrial block, the SA node discharges impulses at regular intervals.

■ Chapter 5

■ Page 67
Cross-training

					¹P		²C	³A	F	F	E	I	N	E
---	---	---	⁴Q	R	S			T						
				E			⁵R	E	G	U	L	⁶A	R	
⁷P				M				I				B		
A	⁸C			A				A				O		
U	A			T				L				V		
S	T			U								E		
⁹E	L	E	C	T	R	O	L	Y	T	E				
	C			E									
	H												
	¹⁰O	U	T	S	I	D	E			¹¹O			
	L									R			
	¹²A	U	T	O	M	A	T	I	C	I	T	Y		
	M							G					
	I							I					
	N		¹³B	I	G	E	M	I	N	Y			
	E												

■ Page 68

Boxing match

2. sinoatrial, 3. reentry, 4. ectopic, 5. atrial kick, 6. automaticity, 7. conduction, 8. pacemaker, 9. repolarization, 10. tachycardia

■ Page 69

You make the call

- Rhythm: Atrial and ventricular rhythms are irregular
- Rate: Atrial and ventricular rates are each 90 beats/minute
- P wave: Abnormal with PAC; some lost in previous T wave
- PR interval: 0.20 second
- QRS complex: 0.08 second
- T wave: Abnormal with some embedded P waves
- QT interval: 0.32 second
- Other: Noncompensatory pause
- Arrhythmia: Premature atrial contractions

■ Page 70

Strike out

1. ~~Three or more successive ectopic atrial beats at a rate of 100 to 120 beats/minute characterize atrial tachycardia.~~ Atrial tachycardia is characterized by three or more successive ectopic atrial beats at a rate of 140 to 250 beats/minute.
3. ~~Hyperthyroidism is the most common cause of atrial tachycardia.~~ Digoxin toxicity is the most common cause of atrial tachycardia.
4. ~~A decrease in myocardial consumption and an increase in oxygen supply result from atrial tachycardia.~~ The rapid rate associated with atrial tachycardia shortens diastole, resulting in a loss of atrial kick, reduced cardiac output, reduced coronary perfusion, and ischemic myocardial changes.

Power stretch

1. D, E, G
2. B, F, H
3. A, C
- Rhythm strip 1: Multifocal atrial tachycardia
- Rhythm strip 2: Paroxysmal atrial tachycardia
- Rhythm strip 3: Atrial tachycardia with 2:1 block

■ Page 71

You make the call

- Rhythm: Atrial and ventricular rhythms are regular
- Rate: Atrial and ventricular rates are each 210 beats/minute
- P wave: Almost hidden in T wave
- PR interval: 0.12 second
- QRS complex: 0.10 second
- T wave: Distorted by P wave
- QT interval: 0.20 second
- Other: None
- Arrhythmia: Atrial tachycardia

Page 72
Fair or foul?

1. Hypotension
4. Yellow-green halos around visual images
5. Hallucinations
6. Vomiting

You make the call

Answer: Carotid sinus massage may be used to diagnose atrial tachycardias. Massaging the carotid sinus stimulates the vagus nerve, which then inhibits firing of the sinoatrial (SA) node and slows atrioventricular node conduction. As a result, the SA node can resume its job as primary pacemaker.

Page 73
Hit or miss

1. False. In atrial tachycardia, the ventricular rhythm is regular when the block is constant and irregular when it isn't.
2. False. A patient with PAT may complain about a sudden fast heartbeat or palpitations.
3. True.
4. True.
5. False. In patients with impaired left ventricular function, these drugs are contraindicated.

Fair or foul?

1. Rhythm: ~~Atrial irregular; ventricular regular~~; Correct answer: <u>atrial regular; ventricular irregular</u>
2. Rate: Atrial 280 beats/minute; ventricular 60 beats/minute
3. P wave: Classic saw-toothed appearance
4. PR interval: ~~Identical for each cycle~~; Correct answer: <u>Unmeasurable</u>
5. QRS complex: 0.08 second
6. T wave: ~~Abnormal with some embedded P waves~~; Correct answer: <u>Unidentifiable</u>
7. QT interval: Unidentifiable
8. Other: None

Page 74
Strike out

2. ~~Synchronized cardioversion should never be used on a patient with atrial flutter~~. Synchronized cardioversion may be used on a patient who has atrial flutter with normal heart function.
3. ~~Atrial flutter is characterized by abnormal T waves that produce a saw-toothed appearance~~. Atrial flutter is characterized by abnormal P waves that produce a saw-toothed appearance.
5. ~~Atrial flutter usually results from an irritable spot, or focus, in the atria that takes over as pacemaker for one or more beats.~~ It originates in a single atrial focus and results from reentry and possibly increased automaticity.

Page 75
Jumble gym

1. **Ar**rhythmia 2. **Re**entry 3. **Fl**utter 4. **P**ulmonary 5. **S**urgery 6. **S**ingle 7. Pul**se**

Answer: Pressures

■ Page 76

Hit or miss

1. True.
2. False. Because the atria are quivering instead of contracting, atrial kick is lost.
3. True.
4. True.
5. False. Synchronized cardioversion generally requires lower energy levels than defibrillation.

Jumble gym

1. Systemic emboli 2. Cardioversion 3. Hypoxia 4. Cardiac output

Answer: Coarse

■ Page 77

Cross-training

					¹Q						
²I	³R	R	E	G	U	L	A	R	L	Y	
	E			I							
	G			V							⁴P
	U			E				⁵P			A
	L	⁶C	A	R	D	⁷I	O	V	E	R	T	E	R
	A				S		R			O
	R			C	⁸K	I	C	K		X
				H		P			Y
	⁹H	I	D	D	E	N		H			S
	I			M		E	¹⁰F		M
	G			I		R		I		A
	H			A		A		N		L
					¹¹F	I	L	T	E	R

■ Page 78

You make the call

- Rhythm: Atrial and ventricular rhythms are irregularly irregular
- Rate: Atrial is indiscernible; ventricular is 130 beats/minute
- P wave: Absent; replaced by fine fibrillatory waves
- PR interval: Indiscernible
- QRS complex: 0.08 second
- T wave: Indiscernible
- QT interval: Unmeasurable
- Other: None
- Arrhythmia: Atrial fibrillation

■ Page 79

Starting lineup

1. Administer anticoagulation therapy.

▼

2. Place one paddle to the right of the upper sternum and one paddle over the fifth or sixth intercostal space at the left anterior axillary line.

▼

3. Synchronize the defibrillator with the R wave on the patient's electrocardiogram.

▼

4. Administer moderate sedation.

▼

5. Call, "All clear," and hold the paddles to the patient's chest until the energy is discharged.

Train your brain

Answer: Carotid sinus massage should not be used on older patients.

■ Page 80

Power stretch

1. C, E, H
2. A, D, F, I
3. B, G
- Rhythm strip 1: Atrial flutter
- Rhythm strip 2: Normal sinus rhythm with PACs
- Rhythm strip 3: Atrial fibrillation

■■
■ Chapter 6

■ Page 84

Batter's box

1. atrioventricular, 2. AV node, 3. bundle of His, 4. sinoatrial node, 5. pacemaker, 6. impulses, 7. block, 8. electrical, 9. cells, 10. AV junction, 11. AV node, 12. impulse, 13. atria, 14. ventricles, 15. pump, 16. blood, 17. lower, 18. right atrium, 19. tricuspid, 20. impulses, 21. depolarized, 22. upward, 23. retrograde, 24. atria, 25. inverted, 26. II, 27. III, 28. aV$_F$

■ Page 85

Hit or miss

1. False. Atrial arrhythmias that are generated by impulses low in the atria may also cause an inverted P wave.
2. True.
3. False. Impulses generated in the junctional area cause retrograde depolarization of the atria.
4. True.

Match point

1. B, 2. A, 3. C

■ Page 86

Strike out

2. ~~An arrhythmia with a PR interval less than 0.12 second originated in the atria.~~ An arrhythmia with a PR interval less than 0.12 second originates in the AV junction.
3. ~~In normal impulse conduction, the SA node slows transmission of the impulse from the atria to the ventricles.~~ In normal impulse conduction, the AV node slows transmission of the impulse.
4. ~~Wolff-Parkinson-White syndrome occurs mainly in older adults.~~ Wolff-Parkinson-White syndrome occurs mainly in young children and in adults ages 20 to 35.

You make the call

- Rhythm: Atrial and ventricular rhythms are irregular
- Rate: Atrial and ventricular rates are each 100 beats/minute
- P wave: Inverted and precedes the QRS complex
- PR interval: 0.14 second for the underlying rhythm and 0.06 second for the PJC
- QRS complex: 0.06 second
- T wave: Normal configuration
- QT interval: 0.36 second
- Other: Pause after PJC
- Arrhythmia: Premature junctional contraction (PJC)

■ Page 87

You make the call

- Rhythm: Atrial and ventricular rhythms are regular
- Rate: Atrial and ventricular rates are each 60 beats/minute
- P wave: Inverted and precedes each QRS complex
- PR interval: 0.10 second
- QRS complex: 0.10 second
- T wave: Normal
- QT interval: 0.44 second
- Other: None
- Arrhythmia: Junctional escape rhythm

Fair or foul?

Causes of junctional escape rhythm include:
1. digoxin toxicity
2. rheumatic heart disease
4. vagal stimulation

■ Page 88

Jumble gym

1. **P**acemake**r** 2. Re**t**r**o**grade 3. **A**utomat**i**city 4. Sy**n**cop**e**

Answer: Atropine

Hit or miss

1. True.
2. True.
3. False. With an accelerated junctional rhythm, the rhythm is regular.
4. True.

■ Page 89

Cross-training

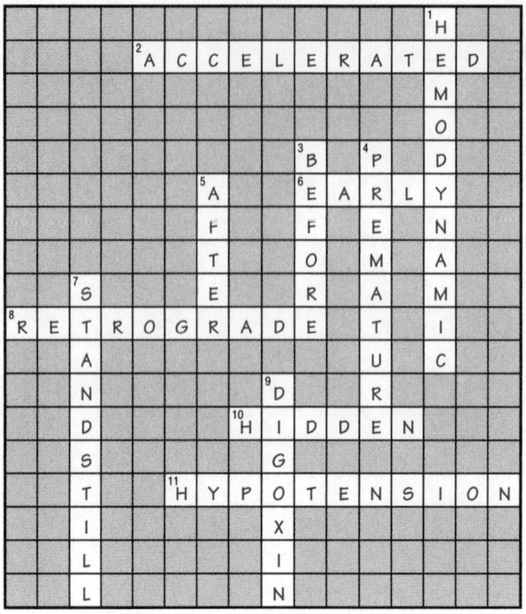

(Completed crossword grid)

Across:
2. ACCELERATED
6. EARLY
8. RETROGRADE
10. HIDDEN
11. HYPOTENSION

Down:
1. HEMODYNAMIC
3. BEFORE
4. PRELIMINARY
5. AFTER
7. STANDSTILL
9. DIGOXIN

■ Page 90

Fair or foul?

1. Rhythm: Regular
2. Rate: ~~100 beats/minute~~ Correct answer: <u>80 beats/minute</u>
3. P wave: ~~Inverted and preceding each QRS complex~~ Correct answer: <u>Absent</u>
4. PR interval: Unmeasurable
5. QRS complex: ~~0.06 second~~ Correct answer: <u>0.10 second</u>
6. T wave: ~~Unidentifiable~~ Correct answer: <u>Normal</u>
7. QT interval: 0.32 second
8. Other: None

■ Page 91

Match point

1. C, 2. D, 3. A, 4. B

Strike out

1. ~~Two PJCs occur in a row in junctional tachycardia.~~ In junctional tachycardia, three or more PJCs occur in a row.
3. ~~A patient with recurrent junctional tachycardia may be treated with cardioversion.~~ A patient with recurrent junctional tachycardia may be treated with ablation therapy followed by a pacemaker insertion.

■ Page 92

You make the call

- Rhythm: Atrial and ventricular rhythms are regular
- Rate: Atrial and ventricular rates are each 115 beats/minute
- P wave: Inverted; follows QRS complex
- PR interval: Unmeasurable
- QRS complex: 0.08 second
- T wave: Normal
- QT interval: 0.36 second
- Other: None
- Arrhythmia: Junctional tachycardia

■ Page 93

Cross-training

Match point

1. D, 2. A, 3. C, 4. B

■ Page 94

Fair or foul?

1. Rhythm: Irregular atrial and ventricular rhythms
2. Rate: Atrial and ventricular rates of ~~80 beats/minute~~ Correct answer: <u>50 beats/minute</u>
3. P wave: Changes in size and shape; first P wave inverted, second upright
4. PR interval: Variable
5. QRS complex: ~~0.10 second~~ Correct answer: <u>0.08 second</u>
6. T wave: Normal
7. QT interval: ~~0.32 second~~ Correct answer: <u>0.44 second</u>
8. Other: None

■ Page 95
You make the call

- Rhythm: Atrial and ventricular rhythms are regular
- Rate: Atrial and ventricular rates are each 47 beats/minute
- P wave: Inverted
- PR interval: 0.08 second
- QRS complex: 0.06 second
- T wave: Normal
- QT interval: 0.42 second
- Other: None
- Arrhythmia: Junctional escape rhythm

■ Page 96
Power stretch

1. Ablation, D
2. Wandering pacemaker, C
3. Inverted, A
4. Junctional arrhythmia, B
5. Delta wave, E
6. Junctional tachycardia, F

■ Page 97
You make the call

- Rhythm: Atrial and ventricular rhythms are regular
- Rate: Atrial and ventricular rates are each 40 beats/minute
- P wave: Normal configuration, except inverted on the second beat
- PR interval: 0.08 second on second beat and 0.16 second on others
- QRS complex: 0.08 second
- T wave: Tall and peaked
- QT interval: 0.48 second
- Other: Second beat conducted early
- Arrhythmia: Sinus bradycardia with PJCs

■ Page 98
Match point

1. B, 2. C, 3. A

Chapter 7

■ Page 102

Batter's box

1. ventricles, 2. bundle of His, 3. depolarize, 4. myocardium, 5. QRS complex, 6. ventricles, 7. T wave, 8. QRS complex, 9. opposite, 10. action potential, 11. depolarization, 12. repolarization, 13. absent, 14. atrial, 15. ventricles, 16. atrial kick, 17. cardiac output, 18. 30%, 19. decompensation, 20. hypotension, 21. angina, 22. syncope, 23. respiratory, 24. cardiac output

■ Page 103

Strike out

2. ~~Premature ventricular contractions rarely lead to more serious arrhythmias.~~ Premature ventricular contractions can lead to more serious arrhythmias, such as ventricular tachycardia or ventricular fibrillation.

4. ~~When a PVC strikes on the upslope of the preceding normal T wave, it's called the R-on-T phenomenon.~~ When a PVC strikes on the downslope of the preceding normal T wave, it's called the R-on-T phenomenon.

Fair or foul?

Conditions that can disrupt electrolyte shifts and cause PVCs include:
2. Metabolic acidosis
3. Digoxin toxicity
4. Enlargement of the ventricular chambers
5. Caffeine or alcohol ingestion

■ Page 104

You make the call

- Rhythm: Atrial and ventricular rhythms are irregular
- Rate: Atrial and ventricular rates are each 120 beats/minute
- P wave: Absent with PVC but present with other QRS complexes
- PR interval: 0.12 second in underlying rhythm
- QRS complex: Early with bizarre configuration and duration of 0.14 second in PVC; 0.08 second in underlying rhythm
- T wave: Normal; opposite direction from QRS complex with PVC
- QT interval: 0.28 second with underlying rhythm
- Other: Underlying rhythm sinus tachycardia; compensatory pause after PVC
- Arrhythmia: Premature ventricular contractions

■ Page 105

Cross-training

												¹H		
												O		
							²W	E	A	K	E	R		
												I		
³D	I	S	⁴T	O	R	T						Z		
			R									O		
		⁵I	S	C	H	E	⁶M	I	C		N		
			G				Y				T		⁷I
⁸L	A	T	E			⁹B	O				A		N
			M			I	¹⁰C	O	U	P	L	E	T
			I			G	A	R					E
			N			E	R						R
			Y			M	D			¹¹U			P
						I	I			N			O
						N	T			I			L
		¹²E	A	R	L	Y	I			F			A
					¹³S	A	L	V	O				T
									R				E
									M				D

■ Page 106

Match point

1. B, 2. D, 3. C, 4. A

■ Page 107

Fair or foul?

- Rhythm: Regular
- Rate: Unable to determine atrial rate; ventricular rate of 35 beats/minute
- P wave: ~~Follows QRS complex~~ Correct answer: <u>Absent</u>
- PR interval: Unmeasurable
- QRS complex: Wide and bizarre
- T wave: ~~Normal~~ Correct answer: <u>Deflection opposite QRS complex</u>
- QT interval: ~~0.30 second~~ Correct answer: <u>0.60 second</u>
- Other: None

Hit or miss

1. True.
2. False. Wide QRS complex tachycardia should be evaluated as regular or irregular. If regular, treat as ventricular tachycardia. If irregular, treat as atrial fibrillation with aberrancy.
3. True.
4. False. Polymorphic ventricular tachycardia has a QRS complex shape that constantly changes.

■ Page 108

You make the call

Answer: This device is a transcutaneous pacemaker. In life-threatening situations in which time is critical, a transcutaneous pacemaker may be used to regulate heart rate. This device sends an electrical impulse from the pulse generator to the heart by way of two electrodes placed on the patient's chest and back.

The electrodes are placed on either side of the heart at heart level so the electrical stimulus has only a short distance to travel. Transcutaneous pacing is quick and effective, but it may be painful. It's used only until transvenous pacing can be started.

Jumble gym

1. Refractory 2. Repolarization 3. Myocardial ischemia 4. Ventricles

Answer: Lidocaine

■ Page 109

Match point

1. B, 2. D, 3. A, 4. C

You make the call

- Rhythm: Atrial and ventricular rhythms are regular
- Rate: Atrial and ventricular rates are each 187 beats/minute
- P wave: Absent
- PR interval: Unmeasurable
- QRS complex: 0.24 second; wide and bizarre
- T wave: Opposite direction of QRS complex
- QT interval: Unmeasurable
- Other: None
- Arrhythmia: Ventricular tachycardia

■ Page 110

Cross-training

■ Page 111
Strike out

2. ~~Ventricular fibrillation should never be treated with such drugs as amiodarone, lidocaine, procainamide, and magnesium sulfate.~~ Drugs, such as amiodarone, lidocaine, procainamide, and magnesium sulfate may be given to a patient with ventricular fibrillation.
3. ~~Smaller (or fine) fibrillatory waves are easier to convert to a normal rhythm than are larger waves.~~ Larger, or coarse, fibrillatory waves are easier to convert to a normal rhythm than are smaller waves because larger waves indicate a greater degree of electrical activity in the heart.

■ Page 112
Fair or foul?

- Rhythm: ~~Irregular~~ Correct answer: <u>Chaotic</u>
- Rate: Undetermined
- P wave: Absent
- PR interval: Unmeasurable
- QRS complex: ~~Wide and bizarre~~ Correct answer: <u>Indiscernible</u>
- T wave: Indiscernible
- QT interval: Unmeasurable
- Other: ~~None~~ Correct answer: <u>Waveform is a wavy line</u>

■ Page 113
Match point

1. B, 2. D, 3. C, 4. E, 5. A

Hit or miss

1. True.
2. True.
3. False. In pulseless electrical activity, the heart muscle loses its ability to contract even though electrical activity is preserved.
4. True.

■ Page 114
Starting lineup

1. Assess airway, breathing, and circulation; then start CPR.

2. Administer epinephrine, 1 mg I.V. push; repeat every 3 to 5 minutes.

3. Consider giving one dose of vasopressin 40 units I.V.

4. Consider atropine, 1 mg I.V.; repeat every 3 to 5 minutes to a maximum of 0.04 mg/kg.

Match point

1. B, 2. A

Chapter 8

Page 118

Batter's box

1. interruption, 2. atria, 3. ventricles, 4. partial, 5. conduction, 6. AV node, 7. bundle of His, 8. bundle branches, 9. SA node, 10. AV node, 11. 60, 12. 100, 13. impulses, 14. ventricular, 15. heart, 16. light-headedness, 17. hypotension, 18. confusion, 19. heart conditions, 20. drugs, 21. cardiac conduction

Page 119

Team up

1. A, 2. A and B, 3. B, 4. A, 5. A, 6. A, 7. B, 8. B, 9. A

Cross-training

¹D	E	L	²A	Y	E	D			
			B				³S		
			L				E		
			A				V		
			T				E		
			I				R		
	⁴M	Y	O	C	A	⁵R	D	I	T	I	⁶S
		N				E	T		S
						G	Y		E
						U			V
					⁷L	O	N	G	R
					A			E
⁸T	E	M	P	O	R	A	R	Y	D

Page 120

Match point

1. C, 2. A, 3. D, 4. B

You make the call

- Rhythm: Atrial and ventricular rhythms are regular
- Rate: Atrial and ventricular rates are each 75 beats/minute
- P wave: Normal
- PR interval: 0.32 second
- QRS complex: 0.08 second
- T wave: Normal
- QT interval: 0.40 second
- Other: PR interval prolonged but constant
- Arrhythmia: First-degree AV block

■ Page 121
Hit or miss

1. True.
2. False. The pattern of grouped beating seen in type I second-degree block is referred to as the footprints of Wenckebach.
3. False. For a symptomatic patient with type I second-degree block, atropine may improve AV node conduction. A temporary pacemaker may be required for long-term relief of symptoms.
4. True.

Jumble gym

1. Asymptomatic 2. Wenckebach 3. Atropine 4. Mobitz

Answer: Hypotension

■ Page 122
Fair or foul?

- Rhythm: Atrial—regular; ventricular—irregular
- Rate: ~~Atrial—100 beats/minute; ventricular—60 beats/minute~~ Correct answer: <u>Atrial—80 beats/minute; ventricular—50 beats/minute</u>
- P wave: Normal
- PR interval: ~~Unmeasurable~~ Correct answer: <u>Progressively prolonged</u>
- QRS complex: 0.08 second
- T wave: ~~Normal~~ Correct answer: <u>Inverted</u>
- QT interval: ~~0.36 second~~ Correct answer: <u>0.46 second</u>
- Other: Wenckebach pattern of grouped beats

■ Page 123
Match point

1. E, 2. A, 3. D, 4. G, 5. B, 6. F, 7. C

■ Page 124
You make the call

- Rhythm: Atrial and ventricular rhythms are regular
- Rate: Atrial is 120 beats/minute; ventricular is 40 beats/minute
- P wave: Normal but some not followed by a QRS complex
- PR interval: 0.16 second
- QRS complex: 0.10 second, periodically absent
- T wave: Slightly peaked
- QT interval: 0.48 second
- Other: Block is 3:1

■ Page 125

Strike out

2. ~~In type II second-degree AV block, if the block is constant, such as 2:1 or 3:1, the rhythm is irregular.~~ If the block is constant in type II second-degree AV block, the rhythm is regular.

3. ~~When two or more successive ventricular impulses are blocked, the conduction disturbance is called high-grade AV block.~~ High-grade AV block refers to the conduction disturbance that results from two or more successive atrial impulses are blocked.

Team up

1. A, 2. B, 3. A, 4. B, 5. B, 6. A

■ Page 126

Fair or foul?

- Rhythm: Atrial—regular; ventricular—irregular
- Rate: ~~Atrial—100 beats/minute; ventricular—60 beats/minute~~ Correct answer: Atrial—60 beats/minute; ventricular—50 beats/minute
- P wave: Normal
- PR interval: ~~Unmeasurable~~ Correct answer: 0.28 second
- QRS complex: 0.10 second
- T wave: Normal
- QT interval: ~~0.45 second~~ Correct answer: 0.60 second
- Other: ~~None~~ Correct answer: PR and R-R intervals are constant before a dropped beat

■ Page 127

Cross-training

■ Page 128
You make the call

- Rhythm: Atrial and ventricular rhythms are regular
- Rate: Atrial is 90 beats/minute; ventricular is 30 beats/minute
- P wave: Normal
- PR interval: Variable
- QRS complex: 0.16 second
- T wave: Normal
- QT interval: 0.56 second
- Other: P waves without QRS complexes
- Arrhythmia: Third-degree AV block

■ Page 129
Team up

1. B, 2. B, 3. A and B, 4. A, 5. B, 6. A and B, 7. A and B, 8. A and B, 9. A and B, 10. A and B

Match point

1. B, 2. A, 3. C

■ Page 130
Match point

1. C; 2. A; 3. B, 4. D

■ Chapter 9

■ Page 134

Boxing match

2. lithium, 3. contraction, 4. electrode, 5. sick sinus, 6. myocardium, 7. myocardial infarction, 8. depolarize, 9. atrioventricular, 10. implanted

Match point

1. B, 2. A, 3. C

■ Page 135

Cross-training

					1				2						3	
					T	R	A	B	E	C	U	L	A	E		T
									A							E
			4						P		5					M
			T								C					
6																
P	E	R	M	A	N	E	N	T		L					P	
	N						U		A		7		8		O	
						R		V		T		E		R		
						9										
					E	P	I	C	A	R	D	I	A	L		
			10				C		N		O		R			
			B													
11																
M	I	L	L	I	V	O	L	T	S		C		Y			
		P				E		V		A						
12																
U	N	I	P	O	L	A	R			E		R				
		L						N		D						
		A						O		I						
13																
C	I	R	C	U	I	T	R	Y		U		U				
										S		M				

■ Page 136

Strike out

2. ~~On an ECG, a pacemaker spike occurs when the pacemaker sends an electrical impulse to the SA node.~~ A pacemaker spike occurs when the pacemaker sends an electrical impulse to the heart muscle.
3. ~~Lead placement for a pacemaker is dependent on the age of the patient.~~ Lead placement for a pacemaker varies according to the patient's specific needs.

Match point

1. C, 2. A, 3. D, 4. B

■ Page 137

Hit or miss

1. True.
2. False. Because AAI pacemakers require a functioning AV node and ventricular conduction, they aren't used in AV block or ventricular bradycardia.
3. False. A VVI pacemaker won't adjust its rate for more active patients. It may be used for sedentary patients.
4. True.
5. True.

Starting lineup

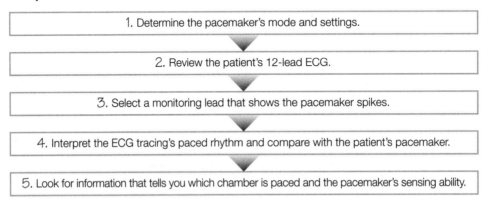

1. Determine the pacemaker's mode and settings.

2. Review the patient's 12-lead ECG.

3. Select a monitoring lead that shows the pacemaker spikes.

4. Interpret the ECG tracing's paced rhythm and compare with the patient's pacemaker.

5. Look for information that tells you which chamber is paced and the pacemaker's sensing ability.

■ Page 138

Team up

1. C, 2. A, B, and C, 3. C, 4. A, 5. A , B, and C

You make the call

1. Failure to capture—indicated on an ECG by a pacemaker spike without the appropriate atrial or ventricular response—a spike without a complex. Causes include acidosis, an electrolyte imbalance, fibrosis, an incorrect lead position, a low milliampere setting, depletion of the battery, a broken or cracked leadwire, or perforation of the leadwire through the myocardium.
2. Failure to pace—indicated by no pacemaker activity on an ECG. Causes include battery or circuit failure, cracked or broken leads, or interference between atrial and ventricular sensing in a dual-chambered pacemaker.
3. Failure to sense intrinsic beats—indicated by a pacemaker spike when intrinsic cardiac activity is already present. Causes include electrolyte imbalances, disconnection or dislodgment of a lead, improper lead placement, increased sensing threshold from edema or fibrosis at the electrode tip, drug interactions, or a depleted or dead pacemaker battery.

■ Page 139

Strike out

1. ~~Biventricular pacemakers have two leads: one to pace the right atrium and one to pace the right ventricle.~~ Biventricular pacemakers have three leads: one to pace the right atrium, one to pace the right ventricle, and one to pace the left ventricle.
4. ~~The electrode tip for the right ventricle is placed in the coronary sinus to a branch of the inferior cardiac vein.~~ The electrode tip for the left ventricle is placed in the coronary sinus to a branch of the inferior cardiac vein.

Page 140

Cross-training

```
     1F       2P            3P
     I    A        4S    U
     B    C        O    L
     R    E    5F   N    M
     I    M  6H E M A T O M A
     L    A    M   R   N      7I
     L    K    O   A   A      D
    8C A T H E T E R   9S T R O K E
     T    R    A       Y      N
     I    R  10B L O C K      T
     O    A                   I
  11L E N G T H Y             F
              12R E E N T R Y
```

Page 141

Jumble gym

1. Atrial flutter 2. Ventricular tachycardia 3. AV nodal reentry 4. Tachycardia
5. Wolf-Parkinson-White syndrome

Answer: Nodal

Hit or miss

1. False. A patient with an ICD experiencing cardiac arrest should be treated with CPR and advanced cardiac life support.
2. True.
3. False. Signs of a perforated ventricle include persistent hiccups, distant heart sounds, pulsus paradoxus, hypotension accompanied by narrow pulse pressure, increased venous pressure, distended jugular veins, cyanosis, decreased urine output, restlessness, and complaints of fullness in the chest.
4. True.

Page 142

Match point

1. C, 2. A, 3. B, 4. D

Finish line

1. **Polar markings:** Identify positive and negative terminals
2. **Pace meter:** Registers every pacing stimulus delivered to the heart
3. **Rate control:** Sets the number of pulses to be given each minute
4. **Sensitivity control:** Adjusts pacemaker sensitivity to the patient's heart rate
5. **Connector terminals:** Hold the leads
6. **Sensing meter:** Registers every time an intrinsic depolarization is recognized
7. **Output control:** Determines the amount of electricity sent to the heart
8. **On-off switch:** Activates the pulse generator
9. **Battery compartment:** Holds the alkaline batteries

■■
■ Chapter 10

■ Page 146
Match point

1. C, 2. D, 3. A, 4. B

Hit or miss

1. True.
2. True.
3. False. Adverse cardiovascular effects of quinidine include hypotension, tachycardia, VT, electrocardiogram changes, polymorphic VT, AV block, and heart failure.
4. False. Quinidine should be avoided in patients with second- or third-degree AV block who don't have pacemakers.
5. True.

■ Page 147
Jumble gym

1. **N**ausea 2. Br**a**dycardia 3. **A**systole 4. Hy**p**otension

Answer: NAPA

Strike out

1. ~~Class 1b antiarrhythmics are effective in suppressing supraventricular arrhythmias.~~ Class 1b antiarrhythmics are effective in suppressing ventricular ectopy but aren't used with supraventricular arrhythmias.
3. ~~Lidocaine is the drug of choice in suppressing ventricular arrhythmias.~~ Lidocaine was once the drug of choice for suppressing ventricular arrhythmias; however, amiodarone is now favored.

Memory jogger

- Class I: **S**odium
- Class II: **B**eta-adrenergic receptors
- Class III: **P**otassium
- Class IV: **C**alcium

■ Page 148
Cross-training

Crossword solution (across/down answers):

```
                              1C
              2R Y T H M O L   O
3S                             N
4L  I  V  E  R                 D
 O                             U
5W  I  D  6E  N  I  N  G       C
          L                    T
          E   7W 8A R F A R I N
          C      N             O
     9S   T      E    10F      N
      O   R      M     A
     11D  R  O  W  S  I  N  E  S  S
      I   L      A     T
      U   Y
      M  12T  A  M  B  O  C  O  R
          E
```

■ Page 149
Match point

1. C, 2. A, 3. B, 4. D

Hit or miss

1. True.
2. True.
3. False. Beta$_1$ receptors increase heart rate, contractility, and conductivity.
4. False. Beta-adrenergic blockers block beta receptors in the sympathetic nervous system.

■ Page 150
Mind sprints

Adverse effects of beta adrenergic blockers include:
- Cardiovascular—bradycardia, hypotension, AV block, heart failure, chest pain, palpitations
- Central nervous system—insomnia, syncope, depression, emotional lability, fatigue, headache, dizziness, lethargy, vivid dreams, hallucinations, light-headedness
- Respiratory—dyspnea, bronchospasm
- Hematologic—thrombocytopenia, agranulocytosis, altered blood sugar levels
- Integumentary—rash

Team up

1. Ib, 2. II, 3. Ia, 4. Ib and II, 5. Ia, 6. II

■ Page 151

Power stretch

1. B, D
2. D
3. A, B, D
4. A, C

- Rhythm strip 1: Class II
- Rhythm strip 2: Class 1c
- Rhythm strip 3: Class 1a
- Rhythm strip 4: Class 1b

■ Page 152

Strike out

1. ~~Long-term dofetilide therapy is associated with vision disturbances.~~ Long-term amiodarone oral therapy is associated with vision disturbances.
4. ~~Ibutilide fumarate shouldn't be administered at the same time or within 4 hours of class 1b antiarrhythmics.~~ Ibutilide fumarate shouldn't be administered at the same time or within 4 hours of class Ia or other class III antiarrhythmics.

Mind sprints

1. Monitor the patient's vital signs, ECG, and respiratory status.
2. Monitor laboratory test results, such as electrolyte levels, liver function studies, thyroid function studies, pulmonary function studies, and chest X-rays.
3. Check for signs of digoxin toxicity or increased prothrombin time.
4. Remember that amiodarone should be avoided in patients with hypersensitivity to the drug, cardiogenic shock, marked sinus bradycardia, and second- or third-degree AV block without a pacemaker.
5. Be aware that the drug has a long half-life (56 days) and therefore takes a long time to reach therapeutic levels and to be cleared by the body.
6. Know that amiodarone may increase theophylline (Theo-Dur) levels in patients taking theophylline. Monitor the patient for signs of theophylline toxicity.
7. Be aware that amiodarone may increase phenytoin (Dilantin) levels. Monitor phenytoin levels closely.
8. Instruct the patient to wear sunscreen and protective clothing to avoid photosensitivity reactions.
9. Recommend that the patient have yearly ophthalmic examinations.
10. Administer the I.V. drug through a central venous catheter to avoid phlebitis.

■ Page 153

Jumble gym

1. Refractory period 2. Hypertension 3. Verapamil 4. Calcium

Answer: Elderly

■ Page 154

Hit or miss

1. False. Atropine is used to treat symptom-producing bradycardia and asystole.
2. True.
3. False. Digoxin strengthens myocardial contraction.
4. True.
5. True.

Team up

1. Class IV, 2. Class III, 3. Class IV, 4. Class III, 5. Class III, 6. Class IV

■ Page 155

Cross-training

■ Page 156

Power stretch

1. C, I, J
2. D, F, H
3. A, B, E, G
- Rhythm strip 1: Class IV
- Rhythm strip 2: Digoxin
- Rhythm strip 3: Class III

▪ Chapter 11

▪ Page 159
Batter's box

1. pathologic, 2. angina, 3. myocardial infarction, 4. rhythm strip, 5. ventricular, 6. history, 7. physical, 8. laboratory, 9. medication, 10. telephone, 11. transtelephonic, 12. home, 13. electrodes, 14. extremities, 15. chest, 16. bipolar, 17. unipolar, 18. precordial, 19. views

▪ Page 160
Strike out

1. ~~Waveforms obtained from each lead vary depending on the location of the lead in relation to the wave of depolarization passing through the epicardium.~~ Waveforms obtained from each lead vary depending on the location of the lead in relation to the wave of depolarization passing through the myocardium.
2. ~~The six limb leads record electrical activity in the heart's horizontal plane.~~ The six limb leads record electrical activity in the heart's frontal plane.

Cross-training

								¹P					
					²T		E						
					R		R						
					³A	X	I	S			⁴H		
					N		C				Y		
			⁵Q	R	S		A				P		
					V		R				E		
	⁶V				E	⁷D	O	W	N	W	A	R	D
⁸I	N	F	E	R	I	O	R				T		
	C				S	T					R		
	T				E	I					O		
	O					S					P		
	⁹F	R	O	N	T	A	L				H		
	S										Y		

■ Page 161
Finish line

1. aV_R, 2. III, 3. aV_F, 4. II, 5. I, 6. aV_L

Match point

1. D, 2. A, 3. C, 4. E, 5. B

■ Page 162
Finish line

1. V_1—septal wall, 2. V_2—septal wall, 3. V_3—anterior wall, 4. V_4—anterior wall, 5. V_5—lateral wall, 6. V_6—lateral wall

Hit or miss

1. False. Obtaining a 12-lead ECG takes about 10 minutes.
2. True.
3. False. Electrodes should be placed on spots that are flat and fleshy, not muscular or bony.
4. True.

■ Page 163
Match point

1. D, 2. C, 3. F, 4. E, 5. A, 6. B

Finish line

1. V_{6R}
2. V_{5R}
3. V_{4R}
4. V_{2R}
5. V_{1R}
6. V_{3R}

■ Page 164

Finish line

1. V_6
2. V_7
3. V_8
4. V_9

Mind sprints

- Myocardial infarction
- Arrhythmias
- Heart chamber enlargement
- Digoxin or other drug toxicity
- Electrolyte imbalances
- Pulmonary embolism
- Pericarditis
- Hypothermia

■ Page 165

Strike out

2. ~~Leads V_{7R}, V_{8R}, and V_{9R} provide information on the right anterior area of the heart.~~ The right-sided posterior leads (V_{7R}, V_{8R}, and V_{9R}) provide information on the right posterior area of the heart.

4. ~~A right chest lead ECG may be ordered to identify damage to the right atria.~~ A right chest lead ECG reveals right ventricular damage.

Jumble gym

1. limb lead 2. posterior 3. intercostal space 4. precordial 5. electrodes 6. waveform

Answer: Left ventricle

■ Pages 166 and 167

You make the call

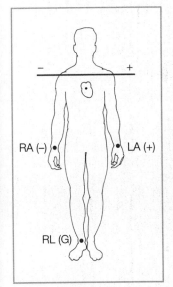

Lead I: This lead connects the right arm (negative pole) with the left arm (positive pole).

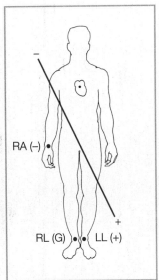

Lead II: This lead connects the right arm (negative pole) with the left leg (positive pole).

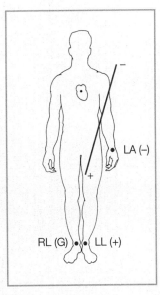

Lead III: This lead connects the left arm (negative pole) with the left leg (positive pole).

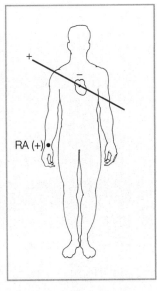

Lead aV$_R$: This lead connects the right arm (positive pole) with the heart (negative pole).

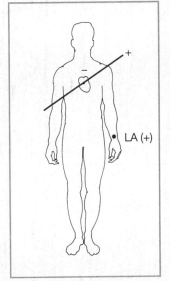

Lead aV$_L$: This lead connects the left arm (positive pole) with the heart (negative pole).

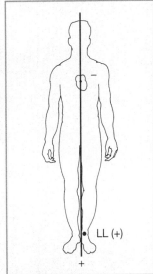

Lead aV$_F$: This lead connects the left leg (positive pole) with the heart (negative pole).

■ **Page 168**

Cross-training

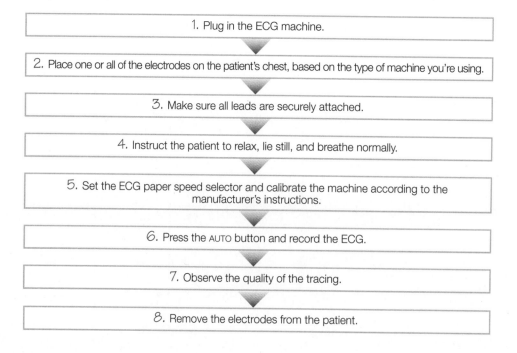

■ **Page 169**

Starting lineup

1. Plug in the ECG machine.

2. Place one or all of the electrodes on the patient's chest, based on the type of machine you're using.

3. Make sure all leads are securely attached.

4. Instruct the patient to relax, lie still, and breathe normally.

5. Set the ECG paper speed selector and calibrate the machine according to the manufacturer's instructions.

6. Press the AUTO button and record the ECG.

7. Observe the quality of the tracing.

8. Remove the electrodes from the patient.

Hit or miss

1. False. The signal-averaged ECG identifies patients at risk for sudden death from sustained ventricular tachycardia.
2. True.
3. False. Three specialized leads are used in a signal-averaged ECG.
4. False. Electrical potentials are tiny impulses that follow normal depolarization.

■ **Page 170**

Finish line

1. Y–, 2. Z+, 3. X+, 4. Y+, 5. G, 6. X–

Match point

1. B, 2. C, 3. D, 4. A

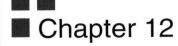

Chapter 12

■ **Page 173**

Starting lineup

| 1. Check the ECG tracing to see if it's technically correct. Make sure the baseline is free from electrical interference and drift. |

| 2. Scan limb leads I, II, and III. |

| 3. Locate the lead markers on the waveform. |

| 4. Check the standardization markings to make sure all leads were recorded with the ECG machine's amplitude at the same setting. |

| 5. Assess the heart rate and rhythm. |

| 6. Determine the electrical axis. |

| 7. Examine limb leads I, II, and III. |

| 8. Examine limb leads aV_L, aV_F, and aV_R. |

| 9. Examine the R wave in the precordial leads. |

| 10. Examine the S wave. |

■ Page 174
Cross-training

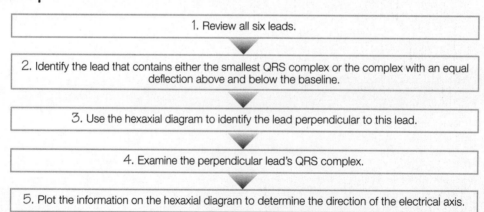

■ Page 175
Hit or miss

1. False. The quadrant method is a fast, easy way to plot the heart's axis. The degree method offers a more precise axis calculation.
2. False. Left axis deviation exists if lead I is upright and lead aV_F points down.
3. True.
4. False. The electrical axis is normal if the QRS-complex deflection is positive or upright in both leads.

Starting lineup

1. Review all six leads.

2. Identify the lead that contains either the smallest QRS complex or the complex with an equal deflection above and below the baseline.

3. Use the hexaxial diagram to identify the lead perpendicular to this lead.

4. Examine the perpendicular lead's QRS complex.

5. Plot the information on the hexaxial diagram to determine the direction of the electrical axis.

■ Page 176

You make the call

■ **Step 1:** Identify the lead with the smallest QRS complex or the equiphasic QRS complex. In this example, it's lead III.
■ **Step 2:** Locate the axis for lead III on the hexaxial diagram. Then find the axis perpendicular to it, which is the axis for lead aV$_R$.
■ **Step 3:** Examine the QRS complex in lead aV$_R$, noting whether the deflection is positive or negative. As you can see, the QRS complex for this lead is negative. This tells you that the electric current is moving toward the negative pole of aV$_R$, which, on the hexaxial diagram, is in the right lower quadrant at +30 degrees. So the electrical axis here is normal at +30 degrees.

■ Page 177

Team up

1. R, 2. L, 3. R, 4. L, 5. L, 6. L, 7. R

Strike out

2. ~~Drugs used to treat angina include quinidine, morphine sulfate, and angiotensin-converting enzyme.~~ Drugs used to treat angina include nitrates, beta-adrenergic blockers, calcium channel blockers, and aspirin or glycoprotein IIb/IIIa inhibitors to reduce platelet aggregation.
3. ~~Stable angina is unpredictable and worsens over time.~~ Stable angina is triggered by exertion or stress and is usually relieved by rest, whereas unstable angina usually wakes the patient, is unpredictable, and worsens over time.
5. ~~If an angina episode lasts close to 10 minutes, it's more likely that the pain is from an MI.~~ The closer to 30 minutes the anginal pain lasts, the more likely the pain is from an MI rather than angina.

■ Page 178

Match point

1. E, 2. C, 3. B, 4. D, 5. A

Team up

1. R, 2. L, 3. L, 4. R, 5. L, 6. L, 7. R, 8. R, 9. L

■ Page 179

Cross-training

Crossword puzzle answers:

1 (down) S E Q U E N T I A L L Y S I S
2 (down) P O S T I T I V I T Y
3 (across) P R I M E
4 (down) R A T U E N T I T Y
5 (down) S L R R E E F
6 (down) S T E N S I S
7 (across) I M P U L S E S
8 (down) R V E
9 (across) H E M I B L O C K
10 (down) W I D E N E D
11 (down) L E F
12 (down) R A B
13 (across) A R T E R Y
14 (across) U N S T A B L E
15 (across) F L E E T I N G

■ Page 180

You make the call

Answer: This 12-lead ECG shows left bundle-branch block. All leads have prolonged QRS complexes. Lead V_6 has a slurred R wave and T-wave inversion. The elevated ST segments and upright T waves in leads V_1 to V_4 are also common in LBBB.

■ Page 181

Jumble gym

1. Le ft ven tricle 2. Is chemi a 3. C hes t pain
4. Infar ctio n

Answer: Necrosis

Hit or miss

1. False. An area of myocardial necrosis is called an infarction.
2. True.
3. True.
4. False. The ST segments return to baseline within a few days to 2 weeks; T wave inversion may persist for several months.
5. True.

■ Page 182
Match point

1. A, 2. C, 3. B, 4. C

■ Page 183
Finish line

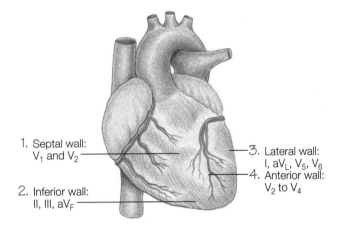

1. Septal wall:
   V_1 and V_2

2. Inferior wall:
   II, III, aV_F

3. Lateral wall:
   I, aV_L, V_5, V_6
4. Anterior wall:
   V_2 to V_4

Fair or foul?

1. Stent placement
3. Intra-aortic balloon pump
5. Coronary artery bypass graft
7. Atherectomy

■ Page 184

Strike out

2. ~~A right ventricular MI is also called a diaphragmatic MI.~~ An inferior wall MI is also called a diaphragmatic MI because the inferior wall of the heart lies over the diaphragm.
4. ~~A lateral wall MI usually accompanies an anterior and posterior wall MI.~~ A lateral wall MI usually accompanies an anterior and inferior wall MI.
5. ~~Identifying an anterior wall MI is difficult without information from the right precordial leads.~~ Identifying a right ventricular MI is difficult without information from the right precordial leads.

Match point

1. C, 2. D, 3. E, 4. B, 5. A

■Page 185

You make the call

Answer: The 12-lead ECG shows an anterior wall MI. The R waves don't progress through the precordial leads. The ST-segment is elevated in leads V_2 and V_3. The reciprocal leads II, III, and aV_F show slight ST-segment depression. Axis deviation is normal at +60 degrees.

■ Page 186

You make the call

Answer: The rsR′ configuration in lead V_1 and the wide S wave in V_6 indicate RBBB.

Notes

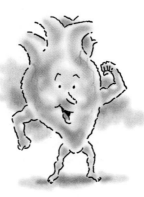

Notes

Notes

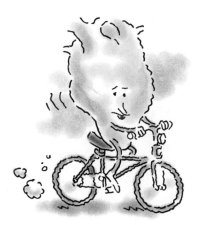

Notes

Notes

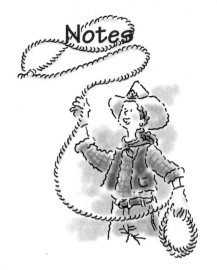

Notes

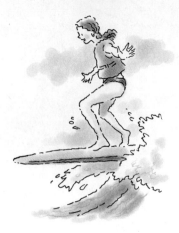

Notes

Notes

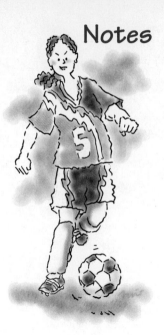

Notes

Notes

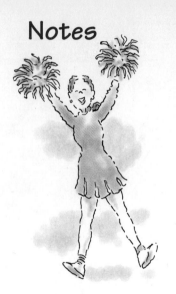